We Need to Talk

Conversations to Ease
Fear and Suffering
Surrounding End of Life

DAVID S. WHITE

Praise for *We Need to Talk*

"The most challenging part of David White's calm, wise guide to the end of life lies not in reading his book, but in opening it. It's human nature to avoid the shadows of our own demise until the last moment, when suitable options are at their scarcest. We all hope for a soft landing; the good medicine of *We Need to Talk* greatly improves one's chances of such an outcome."

— Garry Trudeau

"Here is an insightful wake up call to all of us to shape our end-of-life journey more consciously and deliberately. *We Need to Talk* is a powerful guide to the conversations and decisions that it's time to embrace. David White shows us how."

— Hans Boerma, MD

"David's personal stories and bedside experiences give us a glimpse of what it's like to be at the end of life. These beautifully written accounts, coupled with the practical tips and tools that he provides, give me hope that we can all live well until the end."

— Meghan Maclean, MD, Palliative Care Physician

"An important book about a sacred topic, subtly delivered."

— John Malcomson, Interfaith Chaplain

"*We Need to Talk* is a valuable contribution to our contemporary American culture, encouraging conversations we all need to be having... Weaving powerful stories drawn from his chaplaincy practice, and personal life, White has sewn expert wisdom and contemporary resources into a compelling guide... *We Need to Talk* synthesizes guidance from key thought leaders and offers ready access to useful resources to make planning for the end of life natural, rather than daunting. It's a book to read and give to others."

— Ira Byock, MD, author of *Dying Well* and *The Best Care Possible,* Founder & Senior Vice President for Strategic Innovation, The Institute for Human Caring at Providence

"At Ariadne Labs, our Serious Illness Care Program envisions that every person affected by serious illness will be known and cared for on their own terms. This comprehensive book is a powerful tool in service of that vision... For those who are ready, it's a resource that will serve them well. For those who don't feel quite ready, I hope they'll buy it anyway and set it in a place where they'll pick it up in good time... This is an exceptional book, and I don't say that lightly."

— Erik Fromme, MD, Palliative Care, Dana-Farber Cancer Institute; Senior Scientist, Ariadne Labs; Associate Professor of Medicine, Harvard Medical School, Boston, MA

"David White has written a thorough and eloquent guide, containing useful tools that will assist navigating the difficult journey that all of us will face. I highly recommend this tapestry of well researched topics written using powerful and poignant personal experiences."

— Karl Ahlswede, MD, FACS, Palliative Care Physician

IV   WE NEED TO TALK

We Need to Talk

Conversations to Ease Fear and Suffering Surrounding End of Life

DAVID S. WHITE

Printed and published in the United States of America
by Rose Window Press
www.onemillionpledges.com

ISBN: 979-8-218-00516-0

Library of Congress Control Number: 2022908753

MEDICAL ADVICE DISCLAIMER:

The content of this book is for informational and educational purposes only. No aspect of the contents is intended to substitute for professional medical advice, consultation, diagnosis, or treatment. The author is a spiritual care provider, not a doctor. Always seek the advice of your physician or other qualified health care provider with questions you may have regarding a medical condition or treatment and before undertaking a new health care regimen. Never disregard professional medical advice or delay in seeking it based on something you have read in this book.

Table of Contents

For Further Conversation. The Healthcare
Industry. The Hospital System. Acute Care and
Life-Sustaining Treatment. Conversations with
Clinicians. Palliative Care. Practice Session.

For Further Conversation. Self-Determination. Capacity.
Consent. Advance Care Planning and Advance
Directives. La Crosse, Wisconsin, and *Respecting
Choices*. Palliative Care (Part 2). Practice Session.

For Further Conversation. Pain and Suffering. The
Intensive Care Unit. Needing Help to Breathe. Code
Status. Allow Natural Death / Do Not Resuscitate.
Comfort Measures Only. Palliative Care (Part 3).
Practice Session.

X   WE NEED TO TALK

Foreword

DEATH WILL COME TO ALL OF US. It's a vital and natural phase of life. Yet death is still poorly understood and rarely discussed.

This book aims to remedy that. David White has produced a comprehensive guide for those who want to speak openly and constructively about the end of life. *We Need to Talk* will help you if you're speaking on behalf of a loved one, or if you're the one who needs to talk to your own clinician about the treatment of your illness.

As Chief Medical Officer of the Coalition to Transform Advanced Care (C-TAC) in Washington, DC, I've seen many cases where important conversations were delayed or not held at all. C-TAC's mission is to improve the lives of underserved and under-resourced people impacted by serious illness. And when it comes to open communication among clinicians, patients, and their loved ones, we are all underserved.

David quotes Archimedes, the Greek mathematician and inventor who said, "Give me a lever long enough and a fulcrum on which to place it, and I will move the world." David's book places the lever right where it belongs: in your own two hands.

Only you can choose to use the lever of education and enlightened discussion to move the world of clinical medicine. And it needs to be moved. Too many people spend the last precious days of their lives in intensive care beds because no one spoke up to question whether their treatment would be a benefit or just a burden. And too few people sit down with their loved ones as illness advances to talk about what kind of treatment they would choose near the end of life.

Only when those choices are made clear and conveyed to their doctors can critical treatment decisions be made—decisions that serve the real needs and desires of that person. If the choice is to stay safe and comfortable at home, hospice can help make that happen.

David uses his extensive experience with patients, their loved ones, and members of his own family to show how to make these conversations work. His book will help ensure that the underserved—all of us—will be cared for with compassion when we need it the most.

Brad Stuart, MD
CMO, The Coalition to Transform
Advanced Care (C-TAC)

An Invitation

SINCE 1974, AND THE BIRTH OF HOSPICE CARE IN THE UNITED STATES, a dynamic cultural change has been underway in our nation's approach to end-of-life care. There's been significant progress toward establishing an improved standard of care, yet the work is ongoing. This book's lofty goal is to encourage the next generation of patients, caregivers, and providers to build upon healthcare's hard-earned lessons and growth. Your participation is not only invited, I hope that you'll come to see it's essential.

Your willingness to boldly face this poignant time of life, for your benefit, and for those who care about you, will allow you to author a closing chapter worthy of the intrepid life you've been living.

To accompany and support you through this process, we've established a website with information and resources for your ongoing use at onemillionpledges.com. You're welcome to add your voice to this initiative, and pledge to have The Conversation. Thank you for facing this important task with curiosity, purpose, and abiding trust.

David White

XIV   WE NEED TO TALK

Introduction

ONE BRIGHT MORNING in the summer of 1968, I woke early to comb Nantucket's pristine Madaket Beach. As an exuberant twelve-year-old I hurried along, embraced by the open Atlantic to the south and gracefully sculpted dunes to the north. All appeared to be in its rightful place.

Ahead of me, standing in the waving beach grass, were two people with their heads down and arms crossed. One looked up, pointing toward town. Approaching with innocent curiosity, I felt an odd quickening. And there he was, sleeping peacefully, an old man with his arm under his head for a pillow, the morning dew beaded upon his moth-eaten sweater. It was strange that he was still resting as people whispered above him. My quizzical look was answered with a hushed reply, "He's dead."

What happened next was life changing. Stepping back, I remember glancing out to sea as my perception shifted. Lifting my gaze to the clear sky, I experienced a bracing union in that moment—to the breeze, to the lapping waves, to the rising sun—which in some inexplicable way, upon seeing my first death, allowed me to glimpse what it is to be present and fully alive. A profound, benevolent force swept through me. I felt a sudden and unexplainable connection to everything I could see, and realized that death is part of life and not to be feared. My faith was born that morning.

Fast forward fifty-odd years to the intensive care unit (ICU) where I work, and to a "Code Blue" being carried out on a skeletal eighty-nine-year-old woman, whose heart and breathing have already stopped. Her bereft son, calling from out-of-state insists that "everything be done," and the traumatized family concedes. To satisfy the family's demands and avoid potential liability, the clinical team goes through the motions, knowing full well their futility.

Dying can be hard work, but the evolution of healthcare over the past fifty years has made it harder than it needs to be. This book attends to undue suffering at the end of life and to straightforward remedies, both personal and collective.

The post-World War II baby boom created a generation of seventy-five million Americans. We're a feisty lot. The "boomers" have grown up with and authored profound innovation across the spectrum of human endeavor. Along with these advances has come the impulse to question authority, feelings of entitlement and a prevailing desire for self-determination. In short, we're inclined to have our say and to leave our mark. Upon this landscape, boomers have begun to confront and reshape the final frontier—the end of life.

This generation continues to wield significant clout. A gravitational pull emanates from our sheer numbers and from lessons learned during the social movements and ideological breakthroughs of the 1960s and 70s. The ability to affect social change is in this generation's DNA. Think of human rights, civil rights, freedom of speech, tuning in, and dropping out.

The desire to live longer and better is a defining characteristic of our times. The "first born" of the boomers turned seventy-five in 2021. The growing number of people now receiving Medicare benefits, along with those aging into benefits, is poised to overwhelm an already stressed healthcare system. Unfortunately, living longer does not always equate to living better. There's a compelling need to transform how we think about and support each other at the end of life. A monumental cultural change is underway, powered by an individual and societal willingness to examine and discuss how we die. The goal: to be better informed of our choices, to live longer when possible, and to die in a manner of our choosing, with dignity, less suffering and more peace of mind.

As a hospital chaplain specializing in hospice and palliative care over the past twenty-five years, I am honored to have you join me in this conversation. The conversation is intended to raise difficult questions and to shed light on a path of less resistance. We'll examine and strive to better understand the systems and settings in which we die. I hope to earn your trust so that together we might face the most personal and essential questions. How will I die? Where? And with whom?

Our American healthcare system is hardwired to keep patients alive at all costs. The healthcare industry profits greatly from caring for the frail and elderly. For some, this works well. For many, the downside is fraught with anguish. Across America, eight out of ten people say they'd prefer to die at home surrounded by loved ones. Instead, nearly the inverse is true. Seventy percent of us are currently dying in hospitals and nursing homes under difficult circumstances.[1]

The gap between what we'd prefer and what we end up with can be a source of resentment and distress for patients, loved ones, and clinicians. By realizing the likelihood that we will not die in a place or by way of our choosing, we have a pivotal opportunity to think ahead, to discuss our goals, values and beliefs and affect the outcome. Why do so many of us die surprised and unready when we have years to prepare? The most humane way to die, whether institutionalized or at home, is to plan for it as we would any significant life event. Beginning where we are. Recruiting help. Then bringing our experience, understanding, and hard-earned wisdom to the task at hand.

There is no better time than now to learn about healthcare's systemic "conveyor belt"[2] and to decide how and when to hop off. There are *Practice Sessions* throughout this book that invite you to participate in the process. Their purpose is to help clarify where you are in the journey and where it is that you'd like to end up. At times, you'll want to put the book down, which is encouraged. Please pick it up again. To read on may require confronting a clever adversary—the illusion that it's too early to address these matters. One of the realities of chaplaincy is witnessing profound suffering that could have been mitigated upstream by more proactive conversation and informed decision-making before death is upon us. A prevailing truth: "It will always seem too early until it's too late." [3]

My ex-wife, Sandy, was diagnosed with metastatic brain cancer in 1993, at thirty-seven years old. Our son, Freeman, was eleven. When our hospice nurse, Annabelle, first came to the door, what I noticed immediately and can still recall was her undivided attention. She brought a lightness of being into the room that gently conveyed *there's no need to be afraid; we'll meet this together*. After a quick "hello," Freeman ran off to play with friends while I stood spellbound, realizing that the most formative chapter of my life was underway. While death was rarely talked about, the abiding tenor of Annabelle's presence that day and for the next three months was one of compassion and acceptance. The hospice team displayed an extraordinary skill set, leading me to quietly wonder as to its source. I wanted to draw from the same well. The impact of Sandy's illness, and how she chose to live and to die, transformed how I experience life and love. Hospice care became my calling and has been since.

The following stories are designed to illustrate the three main settings in which we die: the hospital, the home, and assisted living. The episodes are intended to prompt conversations about what a conscious death can look like for you and for your family. The content that follows each story develops themes raised in each setting. My intent is to provide the language to discuss end of life in terms that are commonly used in contemporary healthcare. Learning the terminology helps navigate the depths and shoals of the modern system.

By focusing on the inevitable, we can identify sources of avoidable suffering and outline reasonable steps to alleviate it. This book is a safe read, though not an easy one. It won't bring you to death's door any sooner.

Do you or a loved one have a serious or life-threatening illness? Please read on. Have you been appointed as a healthcare agent, or do you expect to be? This book will be of support. Perhaps you imagine that you have plenty of time and will reach or exceed the current U.S. life expectancy of eighty-one years for women and seventy-seven years for men.[4] This book is also written for you. Even if death is at your door, there is still time to adjust course.

This book is dedicated with abiding gratitude to the pioneers of the modern hospice movement: Dame Cicely Saunders, Florence Wald, Elizabeth Kubler-Ross, and Balfour Mount. These intrepid clinicians confronted a system of profound neglect at the end of life. In so doing they inspired a global movement of clinicians, patients, and lay practitioners to attend more consciously to our dying.

FOR THIS BOOK TO BE MOST USEFUL:

THROUGHOUT THE CONVERSATION you get to set the pace. You decide when, where and if to participate. You might consider keeping notes in the margins and then sharing the book with your family to instigate important dialogue. Whether you are religious or not, please attempt to maintain an open curiosity about the themes conveyed in the stories. Translate as need be into your own worldview. Following each story are questions *For Further Conversation*, which are an invitation to reflect more personally on key points raised. Please note: the term "end of life," is used throughout this book and generally refers to the final weeks of life.

XXII   WE NEED TO TALK

THE APPOINTMENT IN SAMARRA

(As retold by W. Somerset Maugham)
The speaker is Death [5]

THERE WAS A MERCHANT IN BAGHDAD who sent his servant to market to buy provisions and in a little while the servant came back, white and trembling, and said, "Master, just now when I was in the marketplace I was jostled by a woman in the crowd and when I turned, I saw it was Death that jostled me. She looked at me and made a threatening gesture. Now lend me your horse, and I will ride away from this city and avoid my fate. I will go to Samarra and there Death will not find me." The merchant lent him his horse, and the servant mounted it, and he dug his spurs into its flanks and, as fast as the horse could gallop, he went. Then the merchant went down to the marketplace, and he saw me standing in the crowd and he came to me and said, "Why did you make a threatening gesture to my servant when you saw him this morning?" "That was not a threatening gesture," I said, "it was only a start of surprise. I was astonished to see him in Baghdad, for I had an appointment with him tonight in Samarra."

The
Hospital

Chapter One

Placed by the Gideons

People who are willing to contemplate their aging, vulnerability and mortality often live better lives in old age and illness, and experience better deaths, than those who don't... They get clear eyed about the trajectory of their illnesses, so they can plan. They regard their doctors as consultants, not their bosses...They make peace with the coming of death, and seize the time to forgive, to apologize, and to thank those they love.

— KATY BUTLER, *THE ART OF DYING WELL*

BESIDE THE BED, left waiting in the top drawer, the "Greatest Story Ever Told" continues to guide and comfort weary travelers. Started by three traveling evangelists in 1899, with a current worldwide membership of over 270,000 people, the Gideons International has placed over two billion bibles in hotel rooms, hospitals, and other venues in over 200 countries.

As a hospital chaplain, the "Good Book" is a trusted companion. What I read more often though are the faces of patients and their loved ones in the throes of crisis. I'm familiar with a look of shocked numbness, combined with a steely resolve not to crack under the weight of grief.

At Penn Medicine's flagship hospital in Philadelphia, I noticed a well-dressed woman with that look standing alone before the elevators. She was removing a fresh Kleenex from an elegant black purse.

"Do you need help with directions?"

"No thank you," she replied. "I know where I'm going—I just don't want to go there."

Glancing at the Spiritual Care badge on my lapel, she smiled faintly and looked up at the listing of floors, her face tightening to hold back tears.

"My husband is on the sixth floor, the cancer floor... He's not doing well."

I offered to accompany her. She nodded yes, adding, "He's probably worried and wondering where I am."

Except for the exchange of first names, the elevator ride was quiet. Coming out onto the sixth floor we were met by the smell of antiseptic, overhead fluorescent light, and the intermittent sound of bedside alarms. Passing by the nurses' station, I asked Karen if we could talk for a few minutes. She nodded yes and we paused in an alcove with a large window overlooking the city, just shy of her husband's room.

Karen was tightly wound, her breathing rapid and shallow, as their story tumbled out. They'd come to Penn as a last resort, praying against the odds to find a cure for Norm's fast moving pancreatic cancer. He had endured a month of aggressive chemotherapy and radiation. The effort was intended to give him more time and it had, yet it had taken its toll on them both. The emotional roller coaster and accompanying weariness were part of the bargain. Karen cried openly as she relayed the heart of their story. I listened, leaning in with attention, and touched her shoulder lightly to say what words could not.

"I'm feeling afraid and anxious about what's coming," she said.

"Karen, what are the doctors saying?"

"That the treatments aren't working, and that it's only a matter of time. Norm has such a strong faith... he's accepting it. I'm trying to be brave, but I'm so worried."

"Karen, please take a few slow breaths." She nodded her willingness and, with Kleenex in hand, we breathed slowly together for a moment or two.

Her face relaxed and she sighed. "I wish I could remember to do that more often."

"Karen, would you tell me your deepest fear?"

Lowering her head, she answered with barely a pause—"That Norm will die soon, and I'll be alone, unsure of how to cope."

I paused to feel the truth of it. "That's as real as it gets," I said. "Tell me, are you a woman of faith?"

She lifted her head and, drying her eyes, she nodded yes. "That's what brought us together. It's our strongest bond."

With that, we were quiet for another moment.

"We should go to the room," she said, and led the way.

Norm was sitting up in bed in a single room with no window. Unlike most patients who wore a hospital gown for easy access, Norm had on a clean, black polo shirt. His eyes and face, though tightly sculpted by the ravages of cancer, were bright and animated, quite different from what I had imagined.

"Darling, we have a visitor. One of the chaplains."

"Chaplain, glad to meet you!" he said, extending his hand with a firm salesman's grip. His voice and gaze were steady and true.

"What church are you with?" he asked.

"I'm here most Sundays. I guess you could say the hospital's my church. Quite a congregation isn't it? Otherwise, I'm not attending church right now."

Norm raised his eyebrows, and looked a bit concerned for me. I read his look and met his gaze comfortably.

Not missing a beat, with an inclusive sweep of his hand, he pronounced, "Anyway, it's all church."

I smiled in agreement, wondering if he was for real. After decades of meeting people at the end of their lives, rarely had I met someone who appeared so eager.

"How are you doing with what's going on here?" I asked, motioning to his body.

"It's all been decided. The treatments didn't work. That's that. All part of His plan. Thy will be done.

The palliative care team is on our side and is going to keep me comfortable and get me home. I'm doing fine. Ready to go. Maybe Karen told you that we're both Gideons. Over the past forty years we've personally placed two million bibles!" Reaching to his bedside table, Norm put his hand on a small copy of the New Testament and handed it to me. "Make that two million and one!" he beamed. With a penetrating look he added, "I've done my best to be of service. My body's weak, but my spirit is healthy. If I'm not going to Heaven, no one is." His eyes were bright and reassuring.

I glanced at Karen, who was looking down, shaking her head in apparent disbelief, still blinking back tears. There was a significant dissonance in the room. I asked her what she was feeling.

"This is all happening too fast," she said, pausing to clear her throat. "We're believers, so it's easy to imagine where we're headed, but we're not there yet. I'm just not ready to see him go...or to let him go."

I held her sad gaze a moment and gently added, "I hear you."

Norm's face had softened, making it appear he was recognizing her fear for the first time. Breaking the silence, he cleared his throat and leaned toward her. "You know our love can't die. We will be together again before long."

Then there was another pause and poignant silence. In the quiet of my heart, I prayed for understanding and reconciliation between them. It appeared that Norm's battle and now the revelation of his imminent homecoming had blinded him to Karen's experience.

Watching his face carefully, I saw it dawn on him.

"My dear," he sighed, "I'm afraid I lost track of what you've been going through. We've both been praying to beat this thing. I'm feeling relieved, even joyful to not have to fight anymore, but I've been self-centered," he said. "Can you forgive me?"

Her head had been down, cupped in her hands with her elbows on her knees. She took a slow, deep breath. Lifting her head and smoothing her forehead with her palms, she brushed back her hair and met her husband's gentle countenance. While the path to forgiveness can take years, the act itself can take but a moment.

With a look defying description, she replied, "Thank you, love. Of course, I do."

Norm was discharged two days later, and his care transferred from our in-house palliative team to home hospice. I was told that he lived for another two weeks and died peacefully with Karen at his side.

FOR FURTHER CONVERSATION:

WHETHER YOU'RE RELIGIOUS OR NOT, what speaks to you about Norm and Karen's story? Please take a few minutes to put yourself in either of their places. What thoughts and feelings come up?

Would you be willing to imagine how and where your own life might wind down? What would matter most to you? What role would you expect your family to play?

THE HEALTHCARE INDUSTRY

Give me a lever long enough and a fulcrum on which to place it, and I shall move the world.

—ARCHIMEDES

TO PUT NORM AND KAREN'S EXPERIENCE in context, as well as the stories that follow, an overview of our current National Healthcare System will be helpful. In 2014, The Institute of Medicine (IOM) published its landmark report, "Dying in America." It noted that in the United States, though the cost of end-of-life care is the highest in the world, the outcomes of care are no better, and at times even inferior to those in other industrialized nations. The researchers concluded that patients and families face numerous difficulties navigating our siloed and highly fragmented health care system, particularly when coping with advanced illness.[1]

The cost of healthcare in the United States is astronomical. This immense industry, which spent 3.8 trillion dollars in 2019, accounts for nearly twenty percent of our country's gross domestic product. Our federal government's Medicare system, when considered as a separate entity, would be the fifth largest economy in the world. And yet Medicare accounts for only a third of total healthcare funding. *Fifty percent of all Medicare spending is on patients in the final six months of life.* Even with Medicare's lavish spending, over a half million American families each year file bankruptcy due to medical costs.[2]

It's generally agreed that healthcare is not designed to help us die well. The alleged culprit: perverse incentives and disincentives built into the system's fee-for-service structure. The current model encourages neither coordinated nor efficient care. Driving the aggressive recommendation and use of treatments and services until death, Medicare's financial incentives are unknown to most patients and a veiled mystery even to many providers.[3] The BIG winners are the pharmaceutical industry, the medical insurance industry, the medical equipment industry, and top tier providers, i.e., surgeons and specialists. Patients and their family members are often at a loss, particularly the elderly and infirm, as they struggle to navigate healthcare's maze. Given our fragmented, profit-driven system, comfort and refuge are almost impossible to come by when they're most needed.

According to the Institute of Medicine, generous fee-for-service payments give physicians the incentive to provide intense, numerous, high-cost services, consult multiple subspecialties, and hospitalize patients, even in the final weeks of life. Since referring patients to hospice reduces the income of other providers, the fee-for-service system discourages timely education and less aggressive care. More than forty percent of late enrollments in hospice were preceded by an intensive care unit stay.[4] Our current system fails to prepare us for the most important event.

In keeping with the Institute of Medicine's findings, Dr. Atul Gawande's 2014 bestseller, *Being*

Mortal, challenges the reader and the medical profession to rethink how we care for our most frail and ailing patients. Particularly relevant is Dr. Gawande's noting the relationship between an evolving healthcare system and the places where people die.[5] Prior to World War II, most Americans lacked access to hospital care and professional diagnosis, which led to most deaths occurring at home. As hospital care and life-saving technology advanced through the twentieth century, more people chose to die in the hospital than at home. This is still the case. Yet today, as frail elders and their loved ones weigh the benefits and burdens of dying in the hospital, a sea change is again taking place. The result: hospice and homecare are now involved in over half of all deaths in our country. Gawande writes:

> *A monumental transformation is occurring. In this country and across the globe, people increasingly have an alternative to withering in old age homes and dying in hospitals — and millions of them are seizing the opportunity. But this is an unsettled time. We've begun rejecting the institutionalized version of aging and death, but we've not yet established our new norm. We're caught in a transitional phase... We are going through a societal learning curve, one person at a time.*[6]

I firmly believe that all clinicians are drawn to be of service to their patients, yet our altruistic motivations are too often in conflict with the healthcare system's current financial structure. We are each beholden to rules that govern our workplace. Change is due and is in the works. Whether the restructuring comes from the top down, via legislative changes to Medicare, or from the grassroots level, or both, is ours to determine.

The baby boomers—even the most conservative among them—are uniquely suited to pick up this banner of cultural change. Given this generation's track record of social activism, they can be counted on to question the system and to risk reinventing it. Why would this well-established dynamic be any different at the end of life? I believe Archimedes would agree that this generation is indeed a "lever long enough."

THE HOSPITAL SYSTEM

WHILE FEW PATIENTS RELISH GOING TO THE HOSPITAL, most of us are relieved that such a place exists. In 2020, our country's 6000+ hospitals logged over thirty-six million admissions.[7] Our nation's hospitals hum with a taut readiness. Highly skilled frontline clinicians, whose roles are identified by varying colored scrubs, fight off weariness to meet the pressing demands of each twelve-hour shift. Their efforts to respond, assess, stabilize, and comfort are nothing short of heroic.

Norm and Karen benefitted from the most advanced technology and finest care that modern medicine has to offer. Encouraged by a world-class oncology team, Norm chose aggressive treatment against long odds. Even in defeat, he and Karen were grateful for the care they received. The hospital did what it does best, and what it's hardwired to do—it bought them more time, yet at a tradeoff.

In the face of irreversible illness, the purchase of additional time often has a shadow side. In her compassionate yet chilling book, *Extreme Measures*, Jessica Nutik Zitter, M.D. helped us recognize and take stock of how the hospital's systemic "end-of-life conveyor belt," once entered, can be difficult to step off. From admission to discharge, a well-oiled and highly profitable system is driving the conveyor belt. From her years of experience on the ICU, Dr. Zitter revealed the system's processing and warehousing of our sickest and most vulnerable patients.[8]

The hospital system is deeply patterned and historically structured to provide the most reliable and predictable care possible. Behind-the-scenes decision making is geared not only toward what's best for the patient, but *what's best for the hospital*. As a result, being admitted with advanced illness can leave patients and family members feeling unsure of who's in charge of treatment decisions, and often disempowered and afraid.

Here's where the need for clear communication and shared decision-making is most pressing. Ideally, patients coping with serious illness will still have the clarity to consider their options and make informed decisions. Yet the odds of that are often stacked against us. When a patient can't make decisions, and their family is unsure of what to do, the hospital's default setting is to recommend more tests, more imaging, further treatments and to prolong life whenever possible.

It's important to know that beyond legally required lifesaving treatment on admission, that each of us (or our healthcare agent) has complete say over the care we receive. Yet the hospital can be an intimidating place. Please remember it's still your body, and you're in charge of it. Ultimately, you get to decide when to say, "yes, thank you," "no, thank you," and "enough is enough."

Guidance lies in the wisdom attributed to Sir Francis Bacon: "Knowledge is power." Asking good questions of our doctors and nurses and being better informed can make a world of difference in understanding our options and choosing how best to proceed. Our ability to choose an appropriate level of care, to be clear-eyed, and to find our voice, is Archimedes' fulcrum being eased into place. The "world" of our national healthcare system stands ready to be more patient-led, one person, one patient, and one hospital at a time.

ACUTE CARE AND
LIFE-SUSTAINING TREATMENT

THE CATALYST NEEDED FOR THIS TRANSFORMATION is already in place. It is the prolonged anguish of our loved ones at the end of life, too often on a ventilator in the ICU, which number over 100,000 beds across our country. The voice of change lives in the seventy percent of us who say we want to decline late interventions that cause undue suffering. Even so, our healthcare industry continues to push for and profit from life-sustaining treatment, until a patient or their spokesperson actively and persistently chooses against it.[9]

Here's the inherent conflict. When a condition is not life threatening, our nation's hospitals' ability to treat and to cure is unparalleled, welcomed, and beneficial. However, when a condition is terminal or irreversible, the hospital's acute care, fee-for-service model is reluctant to surrender its grip and slow to offer us less invasive options, such as "comfort measures only," which will be discussed in Chapter 3.

Our death-denying culture does not let go easily. Currently, half of all Americans reaching the end of life are brought by ambulance to a hospital emergency department (ED) in the last month of life, seventy-five percent of whom are then admitted for an extended stay.[10] More than one million emergency calls a year bring these late-stage patients to the hospital, often because their families don't know what else to do or because they are unwilling to accept that death is fast approaching. *Many of these patients and their families are unaware that the end of life is even at hand.* A solution to de-escalating the overuse of treatment near end of life begins with earlier conversations between us, our primary care doctor(s), and our loved ones. This could avoid the physical and emotional trauma of a late-stage transport to the emergency department and the likelihood of aggressive treatment.

In the event of an emergency department visit, it's important for the hospital to know whether we have an advance directive, and how our current condition might affect our "Code Status," also to be discussed in Chapter 3. Please be aware that in today's hospitals, it's unlikely that we'll know our doctors. Staff doctors, known as hospitalists, are now the face of acute care medicine. They are often relatively young, culturally diverse, and impeccably skilled. They may consult our primary care doctor by phone, but once we've been admitted to the hospital, the hospitalists and in-house clinical team are responsible for coordinating our care. As a refresher, the hospital's key specialists are cardiologists (the heart), intensivists (critical care), nephrologists (the kidneys), neurologists (the brain and spinal cord), oncologists (cancer), and pulmonologists (the lungs and respiratory system).

It's safe to presume that these gifted specialists will recommend additional interventions, often until the bitter end. At the heart of acute care is the hospital's mission to quickly stabilize, treat and prolong life in the event of severe injury or serious illness. Death is the enemy and is kept at bay as long as possible, no matter the cost. Lifesaving measures, for those with hope of recovery, are a godsend, yet for patients with a terminal condition, the burden of intervention and aggressive treatment near the end of life can far outweigh the benefit. What could make a difference here?

As suggested above, be prepared. Statistics show that eighty percent of us should expect to be admitted to the hospital at some point due to serious illness. As we become more familiar with how the hospital and Acute Care function, we'll be able to better advocate for ourselves. During advanced illness, a proven advantage is to have a friend or family member join us at every doctor's appointment and then eventually at bedside. The value of having another person present, who will listen well, can speak up for us and if need be, fight for us, cannot be overstated. When we begin to talk openly with our doctors and loved ones, and share the responsibility for decision-making, we'll be more likely to receive the level of care we'd prefer.

CONVERSATIONS WITH CLINICIANS

KAREN WAS A SIGNIFICANT SUPPORT to Norm in accompanying him to his medical appointments. Most all patients benefit from having a personal advocate in the room. Karen asked good questions and kept a notebook during their visits to write down what seemed important for future reference. Talking with doctors can be intimidating, given their vaulted status in our society and in the healthcare system. How we view our clinicians determines how we talk with them and how we perceive their guidance. An essential shift takes place as we assume more responsibility for shared decision-making and learn to see our doctors as consultants, rather than authority figures.

Today's clinicians are highly knowledgeable and tightly scheduled, yet beneath the white coat is another human being with a caring heart. The good news is that most clinicians have become more patient and family centered. Ideally, important clinical conversations are taking place in a less hurried way, allowing for more transparency and rapport to develop. One key: Listen well, and when it's time to ask questions, be prepared and brave enough to get to the marrow. Hopefully your doctor(s) will follow suit. If need be, it's okay to rephrase your concerns and to ask for more time.

A common barrier to effective planning: Physicians don't routinely initiate end-of-life conversations until late in the course of illness. A doctor's reluctance to broach difficult discussions may prevent them from happening at all. In this event, the clinical team is left to make decisions about our care without adequate information about our wishes.[11] Lack of clear communication about our end-of-life preferences can lead to reduced quality of life, patient anxiety and family distress, additional hospitalizations, a prolonged dying process, and higher costs of care.[12]

The trajectories of most serious illnesses are familiar to our doctors and are quite predictable. By asking them for the truth, we will be better prepared and informed. We can then consent to treatments that make sense to us. As mentioned, in the late stages of advanced illness, many medical tests, treatments, and procedures provide little benefit. In some cases, they may even cause harm. Here are five questions to ask your doctor before ANY test, treatment, or procedure: (1) *Why do I need this test or procedure?* (2) *What are the risks, and will there be side effects?* (3) *Are there simpler, safer options?* (4) *What happens if I don't do anything?* And (5) *How much does it cost?*[13]

Outside of the palliative care field, I'm told that many physicians feel inadequately trained to initiate discussions about advanced or life-limiting illness. Evidently, clinicians fear undermining the patient's hope as well as being subjected to a patient's strong emotions. In a large study of patients with metastatic lung and colon cancer, the first conversation about end-of-life care took place an average of thirty-three days before death.[14] That's five months after the option of hospice care could have been offered and considered.

The most straightforward approach to alleviate suffering at the end of life is to initiate a "goals of care" conversation with your doctor(s). This type of conversation will be discussed in more detail in Chapter Two.

PALLIATIVE CARE:
"WHAT'S IMPORTANT TO YOU NOW?"

The essential principle of Palliative Care is that each human life has value and meaning... We do our work by learning about the unique hopes and fears of the person in front of us... And then do all we can to be present, to listen, to provide support and to relieve suffering whenever possible.

— DR. DIANE MEIER, FOUNDER AND DIRECTOR EMERITA, THE CENTER TO ADVANCE PALLIATIVE CARE

TO "PALLIATE" IS TO EASE OR TO ALLEVIATE. Dr. Balfour Mount is credited with coining the term "palliative care" in the early 1980s during his morning shower. Palliative care is specialized medical care for people facing serious and chronic illness. The palliative care team focuses on symptom relief, no matter the diagnosis, to improve quality of life for both patient and family. A palliative care consult is appropriate at any time in the course of serious illness and can be requested by the patient's attending physician or by the patient themselves.

The palliative care team may include a physician, nurse practitioner, social worker, chaplain, and other specialists who work together to provide an extra layer of support. All are specially trained to deal with issues that arise during serious illness. The team strives to consider the patient's hopes and fears beyond medical procedures. Palliative care provides relief to both patient and family without having to give up. It can be provided along with curative treatment and is focused on clarifying and preserving what the patient holds most dear.

It's important to understand how Palliative care and hospice care are related and how they differ. Both are committed to the compassionate relief of suffering and improving communication between all parties, while providing holistic care. Palliative care does not focus on death or time limits. Throughout the disease process the palliative care team wants to know: "What's important to you now?" The team's guiding light: to listen, to learn, and to respond accordingly. Eventually, at a self-determined crossroad, a patient may develop the resolve to say to their physician: "No, thank you. I don't want further aggressive treatment. Please just keep me as comfortable as possible." This is when the hospice team is asked to participate. Hospice care is simply palliative care when a cure is no longer possible or being sought. These distinctions will be more fully explored in coming chapters.

If a palliative consult appeals to you, it's OK to ask your doctor or specialist about it. There's no need to wait for your provider to bring it up. Most patients and family members say they wished they'd learned about palliative care sooner. As is all too common, Norm and Karen's oncology team recommended a consult quite late in his illness. In numerous studies, patients who received early palliative care showed significant improvements in their quality of life, in their frame of mind, and even survived twenty-five percent longer than patients with a similar illness.[15]

PRACTICE SESSION:

I INVITE YOU TO "FAST FORWARD" to the end of your life and to imagine how you'd prefer to die. Where would you be? Who would be nearby? Imagine that you have a say in how it will go. You do. To repeat: our willingness to think about this ahead of time and to express our preferences to those we trust is the most straightforward way to alleviate undue suffering at the end of life.

Chapter Two

Crossing Abbey Road

> *When we are no longer able to change the situation,*
> *we are challenged to change ourselves.*

—Victor Frankel, *Man's Search for Meaning*

Malcolm's door was ajar, and I could see him sitting up in bed, headphones on, his body moving slowly to music. The window shade was pulled up behind him, with summer's brilliant light streaming in. He didn't hear me knock, but he noticed movement at the door and waved me in. As he removed the headphones and turned the volume down on his phone, I recognized the familiar coda of "Hey Jude."

He was in his late sixties, wearing flannel pajama bottoms and a worn tee shirt with a familiar image emblazoned across the front: the cover of the famous Beatles album *Sgt. Pepper's Lonely Hearts Club Band*. His hair was unkempt and his face unshaven. By way of introduction, I acknowledged our shared love of The Beatles. He smiled, held my gaze for a moment, and said softly that their music had been the soundtrack of his life.

With his pain under control, Malcolm had been moved from the ICU to a "step down unit" where there would be less noise and equipment to disturb his final days. Only five years earlier he had been on this very floor, recovering from a life-saving liver transplant. Most transplant patients require significant amounts of medication for the rest of their lives to keep their body from rejecting the new organ. Sooner than hoped, Malcolm's body had grown weary of the donor's life-saving gift.

He comfortably talked about his recreational drug use and the hepatitis C that eventually took his liver. His gratitude for the donor and the transplant that had given him these extra years was palpable.

I asked if he was a spiritual man.

"Not so much," he said, with little self-judgment. "I've thought about it for a while and decided that being an atheist is more my speed."

"What led that way, if I can ask?"

"That's easy," he said. "John Lennon." He thought for a moment and recited, "Imagine there's no heaven... No hell below us, above us only sky... Nothing to kill or die for... No religion too."

"What a classic," I chimed in. He agreed with a telling smile and a nod.

I asked about his prognosis. Again, quite comfortably he told me the doctors had suggested several treatments that might prolong his life. He had weighed the benefits of more time and the burden of needing to be closely tethered to the hospital, and he had decided to forego further treatment.

He was referred to the palliative care team, who were helping Malcolm manage his pain and reframe the precious time that he had left. His decision to choose quality of life over longevity led the way.

"I've done everything I wanted to do." he said.

I asked if he'd share some highlights. Number one was visiting England with his sweetheart. "We did Liverpool and a pub crawl tour where the boys first came onto the scene. John and The Quarrymen! It was awesome. We had such a great time we went back the next year," he said. "We joined a tour of Abbey Road Studios, the Beatles' old recording studio in London. At the end, we walked out to the famous crosswalk, where fifty years ago the Boys were photographed strutting across Abbey Road. We followed suit. We were walking on air."

His words drifted into stillness.

Earlier in the visit, Malcolm shared that as his major organs continued to fail and his appetite waned, he had changed his code status from "Full Code" to "Allow Natural Death" (AND), also referred to as "Do Not Resuscitate" (DNR). He reflected a deep weariness but, more importantly, an abiding acceptance that the long and winding road was coming to an end. I gleaned that he might even be curious or eager to find what lay around the bend. I asked him about it.

"I've lived a good life," he said. "I'm not worried." His peace of mind was notable.

Patients often signal verbally or non-verbally when they're ready for a visit to end. I thanked him for trusting me with his story and his truth. I got up and turned to go, stopping halfway to the door. During my clinical pastoral education, my fellow chaplains and I were encouraged not to leave a room without offering a blessing. It's more challenging with an atheist, but with creativity certainly possible. Being an intuitive reader, perhaps you already know what came to mind. Probably what would have come to you as well—wanting to honor what Malcolm held most dear. I offered three immortal words, the title of a Beatles song that's holding up well against the test of time: Let It Be. Through his tears, with the room flooded in light, Malcolm recited the entire song, word for word, each verse resounding with an echo of wisdom and hope.

For further conversation:

Has there been a soundtrack to your life? If so, why not play more of it? What emotions does your favorite music bring up? Joy? Sorrow? Both?

What pinnacle moments can you recall? Use your memory and imagination to rekindle them. What range of emotions are triggered when you revisit your life's finest moments?

SELF-DETERMINATION

COMBINED WITH A GROWING ACCEPTANCE of mortality, patient autonomy or self-governance can be transformational. In 1990, the Patient Self-Determination Act legislated the current ground rules that pertain to end-of-life care. Before this, and prior to the boomers, came the "silent generation," known for traditional values of stability, loyalty, and respect. Humbled by the Great Depression and taught to be seen and not heard, this generation is marked by a desire to work within the system, rather than change it. The boomers, by virtue of the contrasting times in which they came of age, are known to be more outspoken and self-actualizing. Anyone familiar with Maslow's Hierarchy of Needs will recognize this as a developmental achievement.[1]

How does this pertain to approaching the end of life? As death approaches and the medical team musters the courage to say, "There's little more we can do to treat your illness," each of us must choose how to respond. Either actively or passively we choose daily how to live out our lives. The boomers' predisposition toward self-determination can be transformative both personally and across the healthcare system. Each patient is simultaneously a point of leverage in their own family and within the system. On an individual basis, the gradual transition from *I'm not giving up* to *Please help me get ready to go* reflects wisdom and a healthy autonomy. As millions arrive at this crossroad each year, the cumulative impact will force our healthcare system to evolve, to accommodate, and ideally, to become more patient-led through the process.

CAPACITY

IF WE ARE ALERT, ORIENTED, AND CAPABLE of thinking for ourselves, we are expected to decide what
treatments we will consent to. In medical jargon, this
is called having "capacity." At some point during advanced illness, eight of ten patients are not physically
or mentally able to make decisions about their care.[2]
This is when an attending physician will talk with the
patient's healthcare agent or representative and ask,
"What should we do?" This can be one of the most
difficult and stressful questions life ever presents. For
those who have had The Conversation regarding their
wishes, the answer is often clear. For those who haven't
chosen an agent or gone into enough detail regarding
their goals of care, this can be a harrowing time.

If we haven't selected a healthcare agent and
legally empowered them, then the decision falls
to our "next of kin." In descending order, that's a
married spouse, an adult child, and then an adult
sibling. In the absence of one of these, the medical
provider is empowered to provide care, the default
almost always being to prolong life whenever possible, for as long as possible.

While we have the capacity, we each have the
right and the responsibility to determine ahead of
time, or in real-time, what degree of aggressive treatment and/or life support we will accept, and for how
long. When we hesitate to accept this responsibility
and instead defer to family or an institution, we risk
"runaway" treatment that may not reflect our wishes.

CONSENT

THE ETHICAL FOUNDATION of providing all medical care is through informed consent. It's important to remember that every treatment or procedure, except for initial life-saving efforts, are conducted with our consent or with the consent of our healthcare agent. Being clear and well informed about what we're consenting to is of the utmost importance.

The Patient Self-Determination Act was designed to encourage all people to discuss, choose, and document the types and extent of medical care they would want, or not want, when they become unable to speak for themselves. The weak link is that most patients don't fully understand (or perhaps care to understand) the medical care they're consenting to. Most of us trust our doctors to know what they're doing and to fix the problem. This works well until the doctor encounters a problem or terminal condition that can't be fixed.

It is severely compromising and all too common for a patient or their agent to be handed consent forms for aggressive treatment in the throes of a life-threatening emergency. This is the most difficult time to make such a choice. Often, this is unavoidable. Yet clarifying and documenting our goals of care ahead of time can help us navigate such an emergency.

ADVANCE CARE PLANNING AND ADVANCE DIRECTIVES

> *Advance Care Planning is essential to ensure that patients receive care reflecting their values, goals and preferences... A person-centered, family-oriented approach that honors individual preferences and promotes quality of life through the end of life should be a national priority.*
>
> —INSTITUTE OF MEDICINE / *DYING IN AMERICA*

ALIGNED WITH PALLIATIVE MEDICINE, advanced care planning (ACP) is an essential tool in preparing for our final chapters. In the event of serious illness, ACP requires a willingness to converse, to learn about various treatment options, and to express one's goals of care. This process often leads to filling out or updating an Advance Directive, also known as a Living Will. How do we start the process and accomplish this? First, by accepting our responsibility to prepare for such an event, and then by talking with our doctor(s) and loved ones. The desired outcome—making sure that our values and preferences are clearly understood, documented, and readily available to family and care providers as needed.

A concise Advance Directive captures and communicates our goals of care as we progress through serious illness toward end of life. Having an attorney create the document is often counterproductive. Simple, straight-forward paperwork is available free of charge from your doctor, local hospital, or state health department. It's *most important* that, after completing the paperwork, we give signed copies to our primary care doctor, healthcare agent and local hospital.

NOTE WELL: The ability of ACP to guide decision -making at end of life, is not a given. The successful interpretation and application of what we hold most dear rests on the quality of real-time conversation and decision making between us (while we have capacity), our healthcare agent and our doctors. The clearer the conversation(s), the more coherent our care.

THE STORY OF LA CROSSE, WI, AND *RESPECTING CHOICES*

Never doubt that a small group of thoughtful, committed, citizens can change the world. Indeed, it is the only thing that ever has.

—MARGARET MEAD

IN AMERICA TODAY only one in three adults completes an advance directive.[3] It doesn't have to be that way, and the town of La Crosse, Wisconsin proved it. The vision and persistence of a few highly motivated clinicians inspired their community to rise from the lagging national average to nearly full participation. This town of 50,000 people decided to not only talk about their preferences for end-of-life care but to get those preferences in writing.

Here's how they did it.

Individually and collectively, the residents of La Crosse broke one of our culture's most entrenched taboos: discussing death. Through the Gunderson Health System, a team led by Bernard "Bud" Hammes, PhD, and later joined by Linda Briggs, MS, MA, RN, set out to systematically organize a program to instigate conversations about one's preferences at the end of life. What became known as *Respecting Choices* has been heralded both nationally and abroad. The format: to encourage conversations about end-of-life care, effectively document one's preferences, and to make them available to one's doctors and loved ones as needed.

Throughout La Crosse, residents developed a civic pride in subverting the dominant paradigm. In restaurants, bowling alleys, living rooms, and churches, people began to talk openly about dying and to trust that something good would come of it. The outcome was that ninety-six percent of people who die in La Crosse have an advance directive in place.[4] This led to a noticeable reduction of physical and emotional duress for both patients and loved ones at the end of life. In addition, La Crosse has the lowest Medicare expenses in end-of-life care in the entire country.[5]

The citizens of La Crosse proved something important. Completing an advance directive is best undertaken not as an onerous task but as a shared journey between loving family members, supported by community and encouraged by local healthcare professionals. By adding the directive to a patient's electronic medical record, providers across the care continuum have access to the patient's preferences. The net result is that people are living out their lives in a manner of their choosing.

Today, *Respecting Choices'* model of Advance Care Planning is being implemented in 330 US medical centers in 45 states. Respecting Choices' evidence-based programs are helping people prepare to make medical decisions while helping clinicians develop the skills to align care with patient' preferences. In addition, Respecting Choices is expanding their impact by working directly with healthcare and community organizations to redesign systems, so people get care tailored to what matters most.

PALLIATIVE CARE (PART 2)

THE PALLIATIVE TEAM found Malcolm to be agreeable and easy to work with. Some patients are more anxious and afraid. The communication tools to help seriously ill patients discover and share "what matters most" remain the same. The palliative care team at Ariadne Labs in Boston have created a "Serious Illness Conversation Guide" to help clinicians and patients more skillfully navigate these important and often challenging conversations. This guide has proven highly useful in helping people discuss their hopes, fears, and sources of strength during advanced illness. To date, more than 13,500 clinicians have been trained to use the Conversation Guide and more than 300 organizations have implemented it (see Appendices for link). The outcome is that more patients are receiving palliative support earlier in their illness and, as a result, are reporting less anxiety and depression regarding their treatment options.[6]

With a growing public awareness of palliative care and an increasing demand for its services, training tools like Ariadne Labs' guide will allow more clinicians to learn general palliative care principles and to integrate them into common practice. The most basic and universally needed principles are to offer one's undivided attention, meet patients where they are, and perceive and acknowledge what's most important to them.

PRACTICE SESSION:

IF YOU'VE COMPLETED AN ADVANCE DIRECTIVE, well done. You're in the minority. If you haven't, please be honest with yourself. Why not? What would need to change or take place to move in that direction?

For most of us, our reluctance is tied to our fear of death. Just thinking about my death causes emotional pain. Not only are we hardwired to avoid pain, we even steer clear of what we think will cause pain. Given that, it's no wonder that I would put off thinking about death let alone planning for it, for as long as possible. So long, in fact, that many of us die without having made it clear what level of care we'd prefer. Here is an antidote.

Do you remember Charles Dickens's A *Christmas Carol*? What if you courageously allow the ghost of Jacob Marley to lead you to your death bed? Please allow yourself to see and feel the unnecessary suffering of not having prepared for this most personal event. Please see and feel the result of not having made your wishes known, of having given away control, in your most vulnerable hour, to a profit-driven system, which by default will keep you alive at all costs. What would that cost you and your loved ones, physically, emotionally, and financially?

To change this outcome, to weaken and replace your fear with self-determination, begin to focus on the control you'll gain and the relief you'll feel by making your wishes known. Consider and begin to feel the appreciation and gratitude your loved ones will derive from not having to guess, in the pitch of grief, what level of care you would choose. Feel this pleasure and take pride in it.

If you're reading these words, then it's not too late. You have the time needed to take control of that future time, say what you would want and would not want, and enjoy the peace of mind that will come from doing so.

Chapter Three

Traveling the Globe
for a Cure

Despite the billions of dollars that are invested in new technologies in America's finest hospitals, the most important intervention in medicine today happens to be its least technological: timely and comprehensive discussions with patients as they near death.

—ANGELO E. VOLANDES, M.D., *THE CONVERSATION*

MORE THAN A DOZEN immediate family members had flown from Buenos Aires to Miami by private medical jet. Maria, the family's matriarch, had been suffering with Creutzfeldt-Jakob disease, more commonly known as "mad cow" disease.

A leading hospital team in Miami determined nothing more could be done to reverse the fatal prognosis of this rare disease. As Maria slipped in and out of a coma, her husband, Mateo, a successful entrepreneur, was unwilling to accept defeat. The jet's next stop was Philadelphia, followed by ambulance transport to Penn Medicine at 34th and Spruce.

Maria's RN paged me to the intensive care unit to provide spiritual support to Mateo and extended family. As I arrived, Maria's family was milling around outside her room, clustered in small groups. Still dressed in their bright Miami clothes, some stood in silence, while others conversed quietly in Spanish. As I approached, Maria's niece, Lucia, quickly sized me up and brought me into the fold. After brief introductions, still outside the room, Lucia pointed out Mateo at bedside and painted in broad strokes a grievous family portrait of crushed yet unrelenting hope.

"We've traveled the globe for a cure that has not come," she told me. "Mateo is in charge. He is deeply Christian, but it's been impossible for him to accept that this is God's plan."

I looked around the room, making eye contact to acknowledge each person. Maria appeared to be asleep. A ventilator was helping her breathe and she was receiving several medicines by IV pump. The room was digitally and visually monitored from the nurses' station just across the hall. Maria's RN and I traded a nod of recognition and support.

A family member whispered into Mateo's ear that the chaplain had arrived. He looked up and motioned me into the room. We shook hands (pre-Covid) and in broken English he shared his disbelief and shattered dreams. I listened carefully and let him lead the way, allowing for his silence. Turning to Maria, I noticed a large bible, with gold leaf and Spanish writing on the cover, resting under her right hand.

As Mateo paused with a deep sigh, his family circled in the room, and just outside the door, all in rapt attention. Many were crying. My head bowed, I asked Mateo to please tell me where he imagined God was in all this. He looked at me, then to Maria, and placing his hand in the air a few inches above her heart, he whispered "right here."

I nodded in agreement, as our eyes filled with tears.

"Can you let Him lead the way?" I asked gently.

The words would not come, but he touched Maria's right hand and nodded yes.

He asked if I would lead a prayer. I said that I'd be honored to but suggested that he, as the family patriarch and Spanish speaker, would be better suited. He understood and motioned those in the hall to squeeze in. More than twelve of us circled the bed. Clearing his throat and bowing his head, Mateo offered one of the most authentic and loving prayers I've ever experienced. Though little of the Spanish was familiar to me, Lucia later told me that the prayer honored God's hallowed place in Maria's life and so too in the fabric of their family. Mateo thanked God for bringing him Maria, for his success in the world, and for having brought the family this far. What brings me chills to this day was Mateo's plea for forgiveness, a recognition that his stubbornness may have brought undue suffering upon them all. He paused, and straightening his spine, closed with a timeless verse:

> *"For God so loved the world that He gave his only begotten Son, that whoever believes in him should not perish but have eternal life."*

Soon after, still deep in a coma and surrounded by her beloved family, Mateo asked that Maria be transitioned to comfort measures only. With quiet reverence, the respiratory team removed the ventilator, and without its life-giving support, death came quickly.

FOR FURTHER CONVERSATION:

HAVE YOU EVER BEEN AT THE BEDSIDE of someone who was dying? What did you see and experience?

How have such experiences informed you? Given what you've learned, what conditions would you prefer for yourself? Or adamantly not want?

PAIN AND SUFFERING

Pain is inevitable. Suffering is optional.

—HARUKI MURAKAMI

Although the world is full of suffering, it is full also of the overcoming of it.

—HELEN KELLER

ACROSS AMERICA TODAY, millions of patients and family caregivers are coping with suffering that goes beyond physical pain. Pain can be relieved by morphine, but not suffering. Physical pain may be the most visible form of suffering and perhaps the easiest to treat. Emotional, spiritual, and existential suffering can be far more difficult to live with. What is existential suffering? Defined as "being tired of living," it arises when the meaning and value of one's life is in question and no longer clear. Under this heading also is the pain of isolation, separation, and traumatic loss. The best medicine here is the undivided attention of a compassionate friend or loved one.

Searching deeper, what lies at the heart of our suffering and emotional anguish? Isn't it the threat that what I cherish most, my precious self, has a certain end? Herein lies my mortal fear of death, and the very foundation of our death-denying culture. This pervasive fear hinges on the stark realization that my cherished self—which I have established, fortified, and curated over the course of a lifetime—must come to an end. At the heart of my suffering lies the anticipated loss of my precious identity. The elusive antidote: a conscious shift from me, myself, and I, toward a growing curiosity and deepening trust in the great unknown. Reference any renowned religious or spiritual teacher, no matter their tradition, and you will find consensus on this point. The zen master says it quite simply: "No self, no problem."

To further complicate matters, the link between our fear of death and existential suffering, no matter its origins, is intensified by physical pain. At its worst, it can make a person want to die. Every patient deserves to have their physical pain skillfully managed, which has become a recognized palliative care specialty. Its application is an art and a science. The clinician works diligently to find the appropriate medicine and the correct dosage to stay ahead of the pain. It takes time and expertise to get it right.

A core component is that the patient's pain should not have to spike before administering more medicine. Talk with your nurse and doctor to learn about the difference in taking pain medicine as needed (referred to as "PRN") versus by scheduled or "standing order."

With most pain at the end of life, if it's gone then the team is doing a good job. Usually the pain isn't gone; it's being well managed. Often the patient would best continue taking the medicine at regular intervals, plus an added dose, or "bolus," as needed. There's no need to worry about becoming addicted to pain medication during end of life. The common use of morphine in this setting is addressed in Chapter Six under "Hospice Care."

The number of opioid addicts who frequent the hospital have made prescribers very careful about overmedicating. Unfortunately, this systemic caution can sometimes deprive deserving patients of adequate pain relief. An alert family advocate or attentive care provider can make the difference in such a case.

THE INTENSIVE CARE UNIT

A MODERN INTENSIVE CARE unit is a thing to behold. The unit's technological complexity and capability are nothing short of miraculous. And that is the expectation one naturally has of such a place. Supporting recovery after trauma or life-saving surgery is the ICU's claim to fame. Keeping very sick patients alive who are not likely to ever leave the ICU is the unit's shadow side. The narrow threshold between life and death can be a harrowing place. Advanced medical technology can prolong this time of limbo for months and even years. A family member's inability to accept their loved one's impending death can extend this liminal time to a hellish degree. As mentioned earlier, there are over 100,000 intensive care beds in our country. Roughly forty percent of the patients who lie in these beds will not leave the ICU alive.[1]

It's important to grasp that on the intensive care unit, the life support equipment is not only buying the patient more time, but also giving the family time to reconcile, reach consensus, and prepare to let go. Some of the most distraught conversations that I participate in and overhear are the result of poor communication and planning between family members prior to the current hospitalization. If you could see and hear for yourself, just once, the debilitating guilt and remorse that family members struggle with regarding life support, I believe that you'd have The Conversation with your family and complete an advance directive in no time at all.

NEEDING HELP TO BREATHE

ONE OF THE MOST COMMON SIGHTS on the ICU is a ventilator or "vent" pumping oxygen into the lungs to keep a patient alive. The vent is hooked to a tube that goes through the mouth and into the windpipe. The patient can't speak or swallow when the tube is in. I'm told it's very uncomfortable. Medicine is normally prescribed to keep the patient sedated and calm. Often, soft restraints are needed to keep the patient from pulling out the tubes.

A less invasive option, called a BiPAP, is a tight-fitting mask that pushes air into the lungs. The mask fits snugly over the nose and mouth. Most people say that the tight fit hurts. It also makes it difficult to talk. Both modes of support are usually recommended for a short time to recover after surgery or a sudden illness. They will not work as well if your body is shutting down from a long-standing illness, particularly an illness that is no longer responding to treatment. The best time to decide whether to accept a ventilator is prior to an emergency.

Some patients with advanced lung disease choose not to be on machines, but prefer to be kept comfortable, and to allow for a natural death. Morphine and Ativan are commonly used to control shortness of breath, or "air hunger," and the anxiety that can accompany it. An oxygen tube placed at the nose, called a "cannula," is often used as well. Experiment with repositioning the patient to find the most comfortable position. A familiar and calming hospice technique is for the caregiver to match the patient's breathing, while modeling a slow, full breath. Best practice: Keep talking to your doctors and nurses. Ask for guidance and listen well. Please don't overly rely on others' experiences or opinions. Trust your instincts, learn from your current condition and adjust as need be. Discuss, decide, and document your preferences, knowing that they can be updated at any point.

CODE STATUS

IN EVERY PATIENT'S CHART, our code status is clearly noted. The system's default is "full code," meaning everything possible will be done to keep us alive, no matter what. If we're unaware of it or haven't discussed it, we are deemed full code. Advance care planning and the advance directive are designed to help clarify whether a person wishes to choose full code, allow natural death (AND), or comfort measures only (CMO).

The discussion of code status between patient, family and the clinical team is of the utmost importance. It can be time-consuming and emotionally daunting. For these reasons, it is often postponed and even unattended to, often leading to grave and prolonged suffering. If I'm dying and my chart still says "full code," the hospital is legally bound to attempt resuscitation and provide life support at all costs. In this case, the tug-of-war between high-tech life support and the body's natural dying process can be a grievous battle for all concerned.

An antidote: Discuss this with your doctor and healthcare agent and note your preferences in your advance directive. This will guide the medical team in adjusting your code status as your medical condition changes.

ALLOW NATURAL DEATH AND DO NOT RESUSCITATE

"Do not resuscitate," or DNR, means that if you stop breathing or your heart stops—which back in the day was called "death"—no heroic measures will be attempted to bring you back. In many hospitals and end-of-life settings, DNR is being renamed "allow natural death" (AND), because DNR implies that resuscitation is still possible when most often it isn't. The term DNR also carries a negative connotation that something essential is being withheld that would otherwise lead to a positive outcome, which is misleading.

"Allow natural death" has gained acceptance because it honestly describes what takes place when our heart or breathing stops, and resuscitation efforts are not attempted. The success rate of cardiopulmonary resuscitation (CPR), when performed on people nearing their end of life, is less than three percent.[2] In a recent Stanford University survey of 1,400 medical doctors, eighty-eight percent had chosen DNR or AND for themselves.[3] Why? Most likely because medical doctors are best informed about the limited benefits and extensive burdens of resuscitation efforts.

If you can talk and have "capacity," your choices can be updated and communicated to your doctors. Your agent and your advance directive will hold sway only if you lose the capacity to communicate clearly. If your goals of care should change, your advance directive can be updated simply by having a new one signed, witnessed, and distributed.

COMFORT MEASURES ONLY

WHEN THE MEDICAL TEAM CONCEDES there is nothing more they can do to treat an underlying illness, and the patient and family agree to focus on symptom management, then "comfort measures only" (CMO) becomes a saving grace. In choosing comfort measures only, the patient accepts that death is inevitable, though not necessarily imminent. CMO is an official physician's order to stop all curative treatment and to allow death its due. It is an express wish to relieve or minimize all forms of further suffering. While comfort is a foundational goal of palliative care, CMO is the heart of hospice care, which will be discussed in the next chapter.

PALLIATIVE CARE (PART 3)

A palliative approach offers the best chance of maintaining the highest possible quality of life for the longest possible time for those living with advanced serious illness.

—INSTITUTE OF MEDICINE

As THE PUBLIC BECOMES more familiar with palliative care, and its holistic model is incorporated by other specialists, more patients and family members will know to ask for it by name. Note well: Palliative care has never been about "death panels," or "rationing" and deciding when to pull the plug on Grandma. This misinformation campaign was a political and highly effective ruse, designed to stop the Affordable Care Act in 2009. In truth, the objectionable line item eventually removed from the bill was to reimburse clinicians for the time spent discussing advanced care planning with their patients. From palliative care's inception, this moral and ethically based discipline has been about helping people discern what their priorities are, what care they prefer, and how to maintain an acceptable quality of life for as long as possible.

As the boomers continue to age, approximately 10,000 of us are turning sixty-five every day. The growing demand for palliative care already exceeds the current supply of specialty-trained doctors, nurses, and social workers. The current aim is to recruit and train more palliative specialists while advocating for palliative care's core principles to be embraced by other disciplines.

A prevailing challenge: Many physicians believe they lack the time and training to adequately address their patients' psychosocial concerns, particularly those surrounding end-of-life care. Add to that, addressing the family's concerns, and many clinicians just roll their eyes. The unfortunate default is that often doctors are more comfortable focusing their end-of-life discussions on medical terminology, diagnoses, and procedures. Of course, these topics are important to patients, but when a range of other concerns are left unaddressed, there is a significant void for the palliative care team to address.

I see the palliative care model as our healthcare system's moral compass and North Star. This discipline is a brilliant and well-measured response to a pressing and relentless human need to find meaning amidst the ravages of advanced illness. Palliative care is, in fact, the mature fruition of the hospice pioneers' vision to attend more compassionately to the whole person and to "total pain," that which goes beyond the physical. (See Resources in Appendices.)

PRACTICE SESSION:

ARE YOU LIVING WITH ADVANCED ILLNESS? Consider asking your specialist to put in a referral for a palliative care consult. This can happen without interrupting your medical treatments.

At Home

Chapter Four

Please Just Let Me Die

People have concerns besides simply prolonging their lives. Surveys of patients with terminal illness find that their top priorities, in addition to avoiding suffering, include being with family, having the touch of others, being mentally aware, and not becoming a burden to others. Our system of technological medical care has utterly failed to meet these needs, and the cost of this failure is measured in far more than dollars.

—Dr. Atul Gwande, *Being Mortal*

HER PHONE CALL CAME in the middle of night. The call that wakes you from a sound sleep and, even before answering, tells you that something's terribly wrong. It was my mother, Lyn, calling. She had managed to crawl from the bathroom to the phone. She said she was still on the floor, too weak to get up, and bleeding from between her legs. I lived forty-five minutes away, but there was no one closer that she would call in this situation.

"Please come quickly," she said, "I need your help."

"Shouldn't we call 911?" I asked.

"I don't need to go to the hospital, I just need help getting up."

When I arrived, she was back in her bathroom just off the bedroom, sitting on the toilet. She looked pale and drawn but the bleeding had stopped. She said this had happened before but was worse now. She looked frail and afraid. I asked again if she wanted me to call 911 or to drive her to the hospital.

She shook her head. "No, I can handle this."

"What's going on?" I asked.

She recounted going to the doctor, which she was loath to do, about a year earlier.

"I had a routine exam," she said, "but the doctor found a small mass inside of me. It could have been a couple different things, and the doctor wanted to have it biopsied. I said no, thank you, not right now."

"Mom, what were you thinking?"

She was quiet, looking down at the floor toward the stained washcloths pushed into the corner.

As a devoted herbalist, Lyn was predisposed against modern medicine. She stayed far away from doctors and self-diagnosed everything from bronchitis to cancer. I knew that she had been losing weight for some time and looked older. Given her symptoms at the time and reflecting on all that transpired, I believe she had metastatic ovarian cancer. She favored "traditional medicine," and had been using herbs to rid her womb of the mass. In her mind, her efforts had just succeeded. Over the next two months her symptoms proved otherwise.

Eventually my mother knew and accepted that her body was failing. She chose to align with her soul. I can still hear her voice, gently reminding me and reassuring herself that the spirit is eternal. Her workshops with Elizabeth Kubler-Ross in the 1970s had planted seeds that were now bearing fruit. Lyn had relished our conversations over the years about hospice. Time and again, she had clarified that she wanted "no heroic measures" and had updated her advance directive, sending me a hard copy with each change. I had a folder of them. Few words do justice to a parent's request to "please just let me die." We had an agreement.

I called our local hospice for help. Their nurse came out to do an in-home assessment. It had been more than a year since Lyn had seen a doctor, and the nurse was hesitant to call it cancer, though she could see that my mother was gravely ill. "Failure to thrive" was the admitting diagnosis that allowed the agency to prescribe medications, including morphine and fentanyl.

My mother decided when to die. She chose a date on the calendar to stop eating and then a week later to stop drinking. She wrote letters to old friends, decided who would get her modest jewelry and keepsakes, and called her family to say goodbye. Some were not happy with her decision. It didn't matter to her. She was ready to go and was at peace with dying. I think she was eager to experience it, as if it were the next adventure.

Lyn's appetite had waned weeks before, so giving up food was not an effort. A week later, she toasted to life and had her last glass of water. From her research and from accompanying friends on similar journeys, she predicted she would have three days left before losing consciousness. The immediate family visited and said their goodbyes. My two brothers and I slept over for the duration and took turns staying up with her and checking on her through the night. When she became thirsty, we wet her parched lips with a moist washcloth. Hospice had supplied Ativan for anxiety, but Lyn was in good spirits, all things considered. Surrounding her in bed, we cherished the arc of our lives together, a mother and her three sons. We laughed and cried, the four of us, and said the things that matter most. "Thank you...Please forgive me...I forgive you...I love you". [1]

The morning of the 4th day she didn't wake up. She appeared to be sleeping comfortably. We read and sang quietly to her while taking turns holding vigil for three days. Her breathing was not labored; she was slipping away as gradually and peacefully as possible. Finally, her body let go, and she died.

We gave her a sponge bath scented with lavender and dressed her in her favorite clothes. As many Buddhists and others have learned to do, she did not want her body to be disturbed or moved for three days. We opened the windows, allowing Vermont's October air to keep the room cool. People came and went as she lay in wake. A tender reverence filled the home.

In the attic, Lyn had stored a coffin made of sturdy cardboard. Through the changing seasons, while storing blankets or a piece of luggage, I had glanced at it many times. My brothers and I carried her body down the stairs, and then placed her body in the long box. We filled it with flowers, some photographs, and a few of her precious things. We said prayers and then closed the box. We carried it together outside and set it on the cold flagstone terrace. I went in and called the cremation provider, who came quickly. Together we carried her simple coffin to the unmarked panel van. As the van slowly departed, my mother's favorite trees, the towering white pines surrounding her home, swayed in the autumn breeze. Then, with a sigh of relief, a calm settled in.

FOR FURTHER CONVERSATION:

HAVE YOU HAD A PARENT DIE? Perhaps both? What memories and impressions still linger? What did you learn or see that will inform your own end-of-life care? Is there anything your parent(s) experienced that you would never want to repeat? Who will you communicate this to?

CONVERSATIONS WITH FAMILY

The last thing my mom would have wanted was to force me into such bewildering, painful uncertainty about her life and death... If only we had talked about it. And so, I never want to leave the people I love that uneasy and bewildered about my own wishes. It's time for us to talk.

—ELLEN GOODMAN, THE CONVERSATION PROJECT

FAMILY COMMUNICATION AND QUALITY end-of-life care go hand in hand. My brothers and I were fortunate that our mother was inclined to talk about her wishes. We had many a conversation over tea or during a brisk walk. While it's hard to talk about one's death, it's unkind to leave a spouse, a child, or a loved one in a position of uncertainty about something so important. Too many people die in a way they would never want, simply because they didn't talk with the right person about what they would want. The survivors' guilt that can result from not knowing and then questioning whether we made the right decisions is a cruel inheritance.

As mentioned earlier, when family and clinicians focus on these topics, the conversations fall under the heading of advance care planning or one's goals of care. The clear intent: to reflect on the care we'd prefer if we lack the capacity to speak for ourselves, and then to communicate this to our loved ones. The best time to discuss our fears and wishes is sooner than later. "Let's wait and see" is not a winning strategy. Please don't wait until a crisis arises. The hospital is perhaps the least desirable place to have such a conversation. The institution hums with urgency, distress, and the overarching bias of providing additional treatment. Under this gravitational field, it's extremely difficult to discriminate and choose between various medical options, let alone to opt out.

Denial is frequently our default setting in situations of high anxiety and crisis. In such settings, patients and family often lack the mental and emotional clarity to manage strong feelings and difficult decisions. During a traumatic event, we can be hard-pressed to remember our own phone number, let alone to decide whether a loved one should be put on a ventilator or receive a feeding tube. An antidote in this situation is to investigate what's taking place with disarming honesty and emotional fortitude—then to courageously accept the truth, and to talk about it with the appropriate people.

THE HEALTHCARE AGENT / PROXY

NEARLY HALF OF US will need a trusted friend or family member to speak for us at some point during serious illness.[2] Here are two essential tasks: first, to choose an appropriate healthcare agent or "proxy," and second, to have detailed conversations with them about our goals of care. An ideal agent is someone who we can trust to carry out our wishes, and who can shoulder the responsibility to speak for us in emotionally charged situations. Preferably, our agent lives close by or can travel to be at our side. They know us well and understand what's important to us. They will listen well and ask good questions, and will likely be available long into the future. An ideal agent will be able to handle conflicting opinions between family, friends, and medical personnel; and will be a strong advocate in the face of opposition. Just as importantly, our agent needs to know how and when to let go. Note well: These suggestions may lead to choosing a person other than a spouse, son, or daughter, if a more suitable agent is available.

Begin sooner than later to identify and to coach this key person. Your agent may initially feel hesitant to assume responsibility for such important decisions. While this is normal, it needs to be addressed and redirected. In truth, your agent is being empowered by you to communicate your wishes. It is of lasting importance to reaffirm that the patient is the decision-maker. The agent is a spokesperson.

Full disclosure: Emotional after-effects of serving as a healthcare agent are normal and can be expected. In addition to the satisfaction of having been of service, there can also be lingering feelings over the decisions made, including doubt or stress regarding those decisions. Studies clearly show that when an agent has had detailed conversations with the patient and acts on their loved one's requests, any lasting negative effects are minimized.[3]

THE FAMILY SYSTEM

WHEN A PATIENT LACKS CAPACITY or can't speak, even during an operation, their agent or family members must assume significant responsibility. The underlying and long-established patterns in a family's decision-making process (the "family dynamics") can either support or harm the patient. A sole family member's inability or unwillingness to accept a terminal condition can influence the patient's and clinical team's decision-making and lead to prolonged and undue suffering. Some of the most traumatic suffering I've witnessed, for patient, family, and clinicians alike, is when family can't (or won't) agree on when to remove life support from a patient who will not survive without it. The clinical team is duty-bound, whenever possible, to give the family time to resolve their differences, despite the likelihood of moral distress for all concerned.

Be aware that long-standing family dynamics can run the show. During end-of-life care, watch for "the daughter from California" or, if dying on the west coast, "the son from New York." This well-established drama displays the underlying guilt of a distant and less involved family member who flies in at the end of life to impress upon all concerned how important it is "to do everything possible" to save their loved one, regardless of what's stated in the patient's advance directive.

Note well: In most cases, if we're unable to speak for ourselves, our agent has the right to update or change our advance directive as they see fit. Choosing an agent who we trust to understand and carry out our wishes is of paramount importance.

An honest assessment of our family's emotional patterns allows us to establish this understanding ahead of time. The earlier in the disease process the better. If need be, we can even single out and exclude a particular person's involvement through our advance directive.

Another emotionally charged family issue: food and nutrition. Weeks or even months before death, it's normal for a person's eating habits to change. Many family members have difficulty when a loved one wants to eat less, or nothing at all. Providing food and encouraging one to eat is a deep and central component in most every family. As we know, "food is love" and equals nurturing. It's important to find alternative ways to nurture those who, for whatever reasons, have lost their appetite.

In the early stages of illness, prior to hospitalization, it's helpful to keep track of how much the patient is eating and drinking. This can be very useful to the medical team in evaluating the patient's condition as it progresses.

When all a person eats is soft food, such as creamed soups, puddings, or ice cream, they are likely short months from death. Eating no food, they are likely weeks away from dying, and just having sips of water, usually days to short weeks away. No intake of food or water, usually just hours to days.

With end-stage disease, when feeding tubes are

suggested by well-meaning doctors and accepted by well-meaning family members, it can be as much for their emotional comfort as for the patient's well-being. This will be addressed in more detail in Chapter Seven.

CANCER

"The Emperor of All Maladies"

—Dr. Siddhartha Mukherjee's best selling title

After heart disease, cancer is the second leading cause of death in the United States. It accounts for approximately 600,000 deaths a year in the U.S. alone. In 2020, an estimated 1.8 million new cases of cancer were diagnosed. Although we're seeing progress in detection, treatment, and five-year survival rates, fatalities have only declined slowly over the past years. Cancer remains a fearsome adversary.

It's often noted that when one person has cancer, the whole family is affected by it. A strong case can be made that every cancer diagnosis should trigger a goals of care conversation between patient, family, and clinicians. Although "best practices" recommend that conversations about end-of-life preferences take place when the patient is relatively stable, a large cancer survey found that most of these discussions were initiated after hospitalization.[4]

During cancer treatment, clinicians' inadequate disclosure and patients' magical thinking are all too normal. In a study of patients with either metastatic lung or colon cancer, seven out of ten did not understand that chemotherapy was unlikely to cure their cancer.[5] This suggests an ongoing need for clearer communication between oncologists and their patients. A distressing result is that the collateral denial and misunderstanding can make it difficult for patients to consider quality-of-life options such as hospice, even when less aggressive treatment may be well-suited to the patient's goals of care.[6] My intent is not to cast blame but to address an opportunity to improve care and communication.

It's important to ask our doctors for their complete honesty and to understand the trade-off (benefits vs. burdens) of additional rounds of chemotherapy. Yes, time is gained, but quality of life is often surrendered. At what point do we recognize and accept that the treatments aren't working? A brave and decisive question for your oncologist: "Would you be surprised if I died in the next year? Or in the next six months?" At some point, perhaps as the next course of chemo is being recommended, more people are finding the resolve to say, "No thank you, I just want to go home and be with my family and have the best quality of life that I can."

HOSPICE

You matter because you are you, and you matter to the end of your life. We will do all we can not only to help you die peacefully, but also to live until you die.

—DAME CICELY SAUNDERS

THE MODERN HOSPICE MOVEMENT BEGAN in England in 1967, at St. Christopher's Hospital, led gallantly by Dr. Cicely Saunders. In the U.S., this bold experiment in end-of-life care began in 1974 in Branford, Connecticut with the opening of our country's first hospice, led by Florence Wald, Dame Cicely Saunders's dear friend and protege. For nearly fifty years, clinicians have been working to transform our medical system's ability to provide compassionate, holistic care when a cure is no longer possible. The transition from cure to comfort is hospice's calling card. That first year, seventy-five Americans benefitted from hospice care. In 2020, in a broad range of settings in all fifty states, more than 1.6 million people received hospice care provided by over 5500 separate agencies. Just over half of all deaths in the U.S. now occur under hospice care.[7]

The Hospice Benefit, passed in 1982, offers every American at least six months (180+ days) of hospice care, fully paid for by Medicare. For years, the national median length of hospice utilization has ranged from sixteen to twenty days. Why such a discrepancy? Essentially, it's hard to accept that life has run its course. Due to this, hospice is usually called in late and unable to offer its full value. The good news: Learning about hospice and what it has to offer can happen right now.

A referral to hospice is usually initiated by a doctor, nurse, or social worker. A representative from your local hospice agency will normally follow up within twenty-four hours. Providing care in the patient's home is where hospice shines. The explicit intent is for the patient's family and support community to take care of the patient under the hospice team's guidance. Hospice team members will stop in frequently, usually for an hour or so at a time. If you're set on dying at home, plan on getting all the help you can from family, friends, and neighbors.

Be sure to ask your hospice agency for detailed information about what's provided and what isn't. When patients are dissatisfied with hospice, it's often due to unrealistic or inaccurate expectations. Have a clear understanding at the outset what your hospice agency offers, then be firm about getting what you've been promised. Hospice isn't perfect, but it's the gold standard for end-of-life care. Please see a link in the Appendices for an online description of the core services that all hospice agencies are required to provide.

THE VOLUNTARY SUSPENSION OF EATING AND DRINKING (VSED)

> *"I've lived a wonderful life, but it has to end some-time and this is the right time for me. My decision is not about whether I'm going to die—we will all die sooner or later. My decision is about when and how. I don't want to spoil the wonder of my life by dragging it out in decay... Help me find a way."*
>
> —VIRGINIA EDDY, COURTESY OF HER SON,
> DR. DAVID M. EDDY

THE QUIET CHOICE TO DIE through the Voluntary Suspension of Eating and Drinking (VSED) is widely unheard of and rarely discussed. Many consider VSED a form of assisted suicide. To others, it is a sane and viable option at end of life to relieve inconsolable suffering. The topic of VSED carries few established guidelines. Hospices, continuing care facilities and end-of-life specialists struggle to develop and convey useful policies and procedures for VSED. Our health care system is reluctant to acknowledge VSED, let alone to develop and im-plement best practices. The medical, ethical and religious tension underlying VSED exists at the confluence of two mighty forces; the culmination of human suffering at end of life and the default setting of our modern healthcare system to pro-long life at all costs.

What is an appropriate and compassionate response to someone considering VSED? What guidance would help navigate this polarized topic?

While little known to the general population, VSED is increasingly familiar to hospice patients. As end of life approaches, our need for food naturally diminishes. Distinct from this process, VSED is the willful choice of a determined patient. By definition, it is "the action of a competent person who voluntarily and deliberately chooses to stop eating and drinking with the primary intention of hastening death because of the persistence of unacceptable suffering."[8] In essence VSED is death by fasting and while controversial, it is quietly gaining recognition and acceptance. The preceding story, as well as Chapter Seven, describes the process.

For those who choose VSED, common denominators include unrelenting pain, a readiness to die, the desire to preserve control at the end of life, and the desire to die at home. A patient considering VSED needs to be resolute, well informed, and have the support of both their clinical team and an empathetic family or friend group. A growing number of clinicians, including the American Nurses Association, view the decision to hasten death in this manner as the ultimate individual right.[9] It is a quiet choice of last resort.

VSED is legally and ethically permissible in all fifty states. It has been deemed consistent with a patient's right to refuse or forego life sustaining treatments. That said, it's essential for the clinical team to determine that the patient considering

VSED is not living with treatable depression. Every clinician needs to decide how they'll respond to a patient's request to hasten death. Towards this end, medical societies and policymakers are being asked to establish clear institutional guidelines for VSED, and to promote critical and transparent discussion to inform both patients and healthcare professionals. When asked, clinicians who value patient autonomy and shared decision making can include a description of VSED. Others who feel that VSED is morally or ethically wrong may transfer the care of such patients to colleagues who feel differently and could be of support.

Dr. Robert Macauley, ordained Episcopal minister, author and renowned Palliative Care ethicist writes: "If the patient is resolute in proceeding with VSED, there is little that can—or should—be done to stop them. The palliative care clinician is better off respecting the decision and trusting that time will determine whether the patient is truly committed to VSED."[10] In fact, many patients discuss giving up eating and drinking but choose otherwise. Just knowing that VSED exists and could be a viable exit strategy has seen many a patient through a dark night of the soul. For patients who choose to proceed with VSED and have merited their clinical team's medical and psychosocial support, it is *essential* to stop ALL intake, once the fast has begun, *including ice chips.*

For steadfast patients, excellent oral care is paramount during the early stages of the fast when the patient is still awake and most likely thirsty. The frequent use of fresh oral swabs, lip balm, and rinsing of the mouth is encouraged to minimize discomfort. Be sure the patient spits out any and all fluids. As dehydration progresses, the patient will become sleepy and eventually slip into a coma leading to death. While keeping vigil, attentive physical care and pain management need to continue as death approaches.

If a patient's Advance Directive instructs that they maintain the right to give up eating and drinking, yet the patient has lost decision-making capacity, their Agent still has the right and responsibility to advocate for this course of action on the patient's behalf. In her practical guide, *The Art of Dying Well*, Katy Butler offers this cogent directive from her own Living Will:

"I wish to remove all barriers to a natural, peaceful, and timely death... If I'm eating, let me eat what I want, and don't put me on "thickened liquids," even if this increases my risk of pneumonia. Do not force or coax me to eat. Do not authorize a feeding tube for me, even on a trial basis. If one is inserted, please ask for its immediate removal."

NOTEWORTHY: VSED is increasingly utilized by a small percentage of hospice patients who have chosen Medical Aid in Dying (MAiD), but who for various reasons have not received final approval for their lethal prescriptions. Over 70 million adults live in the nine states (plus the District of Columbia) that have legalized MAiD.

Choose a close friend or partner. Stand or sit at arm's length from each other. Take turns asking one another the simple question: "Am I going to die?" Use each other's first names. Maintain eye contact as much as possible. Simply answer, "Yes (first name), you are going to die." Repeat as needed until the full force of this important truth pierces the emotional armor. This practice may open the door to discussing your preferences for end of life.

Chapter 5

To Care for Them Who Have Borne the Battle

LEE RICHMOND WAS A WELL-LOVED and retired college professor of American history. His champion and perennial source of inspiration was Abraham Lincoln. While Lee and his family gradually resigned themselves to hospice care, Lee continued to draw strength and purpose from the immortal closing of Lincoln's second inaugural address:

> *With malice toward none; with charity for all; with firmness in the right, as God gives us to see the right, let us strive on to finish the work we are in; to bind up the nation's wounds; to care for him who shall have borne the battle, and for his widow, and his orphan—to do all which may achieve and cherish a just, and a lasting peace, among ourselves, and with all nations.*

Lee hailed from a long line of Pennsylvania Quakers, who are known for seeking peace by listening for the still, small voice within. Lee was a gentle man, gifted with a sharp mind, yet the acknowledgement of his terminal cancer was testing his spirit. Also, beyond the safe confines of his home, our nation's political and social divisions deepened his dismay. Lee knew too well that history repeats itself and seeing our country bitterly divided was as if the Civil War was raging anew. Lincoln's call for national healing, just 41 days prior to his assassination, served as a moral compass for Lee.

One question of many during the hospice intake process is whether the new patient would like a chaplain to visit. Lee had said yes, allowing me to call on him in the suburban home that he shared with his son, Drew, and daughter-in-law, Jan. Lee greeted me at the front door with a smile that exuded kindness. Walking carefully and leaning on the furniture to avoid falling, Lee welcomed me into a bright living room. He settled into his favorite corner of a well-worn couch. Jan came in from the kitchen, introduced herself with a warm handshake, and brought us water. She sat with us to help Lee feel at ease with our initial visit.

"What kind of support would be most helpful right now?" I asked.

"This is all new for me," he said after a thoughtful pause. "It's hard to wrap my mind around, so I thought it would help to have someone to talk with."

"I'd be honored," I told him. "What would be important for me to know about you?"

And so began a compelling and intimate conversation about Lee's quest to conclude his life's work.

"I knew this time was coming but it feels strange," Lee said, "as if it's happening to somebody else. I'm having a hard time coming to terms with it all."

Lee was a deep and practical thinker, calm and well-spoken. By any measure, it appeared that he had achieved success and was now surrounded by a devoted family. Reinhold Niebuhr's Serenity Prayer came to mind, challenging each of us to discern what we have the power to change, versus what we would do well to accept. Lee's final course of study was to find peace of mind.

I asked if he was familiar with Victor Frankel's *Man's Search for Meaning.*

Nodding yes, he took his cue. "Frankel's central theme was that no matter what may be taken from us, even life, we retain the ability to choose our emotional and spiritual response."

I smiled and nodded yes in full agreement.

"We get to decide the ultimate meaning of what transpires," he added. Lee's train of thought jumped quickly ahead to what would become a recurring theme. "But how much time do you think I have?" he asked. "Is there anything else I should be doing?" It was as if he was prepping for a final exam.

I sensed Jan's quiet presence and her impulse to contribute. Looking to her with a nod of encouragement, she jumped in.

"Dad, I know that accepting hospice has been a hard process. We just want you to be as comfortable as possible and to have as much time together as we can …" Her voice cracked with emotion.

"Thank you," he said with a tender voice. "But I want this to be manageable for you all too," he added.

Lee was alluding to his decision to move to our agency's inpatient hospice unit, just a few miles away, to spare his family the task of full-time caregiving in his final weeks. This is an opportunity few hospice patients have, yet he had clearly weighed his options and had come to a decision. I admired his clarity and self-determination.

When I saw Lee next, he was in a small private room, sitting up in a single bed with "his" Philadelphia Phillies playing baseball on TV. Being it was an "off year," his team was providing only further disappointment. Perhaps that's why he was glad to see me. He muted the TV and showed me a crayon drawing by his twelve-year-old grandson of Lincoln standing before a miniature U.S. capitol, speech in hand. No family member had been spared Lee's devotion to Honest Abe. Choked up with loving pride, Lee appeared to realize that his legacy had been conferred and was intact. I felt happy and relieved for this good man and his family.

A week later, I found Lee about where I had left him, having just finished lunch and iced tea that Jan had brought from home. Lee's expression signaled he had something important on his mind.

"David, I feel ready… but I'm still here." I must have smiled. "No, really, I mean it. I'm ready to go," he said. "Do you think it will be long?" What would Honest Abe have said to him?

"Lee, if Jan keeps bringing you home cooked meals, you're going to be here awhile. And the Phillies are winning again. Truth to tell, very few hospice patients are sitting up, taking nourishment, and talking right before they die."

"Hmm…" he said, taking that in, and then was quiet for a minute. "What would move things along?" he asked.

It was my turn to think.

"You know, Lee, I think your family is cherishing this time with you. They're not quite ready. Would you be willing to do some homework?"

He smiled. "Yes."

"When you're by yourself next, put on your old Quaker hat and listen for that quiet voice. Ask whatever questions are most important to you. Please trust what you find there. I look forward to hearing how it goes."

When I stopped by next, the TV was off. Lee's bedside table was all but clear, no snacks, just a cup of water with plastic straw and, front and center, his grandson's drawing. Lee's eyes were closed, and I sensed a deep change in him, what the hospice folks call "being in transition." The venetian blinds were turned down to shade the bed. He did not wake up. I took the opportunity to say goodbye and to thank him in the quiet of my heart for our time together. I bowed my head, listening to his slow rhythmic breathing, as a lasting peace filled the room. Two days later, in the quiet of the night, with his son and daughter-in-law holding vigil at bedside, Lee slipped away.

WOULD YOU LIKE THERE TO BE a memorial service for you? If not, would your family understand this? If so, who would you prefer to give the eulogy? Have you asked them yet?

Would you consider writing your obituary? If not, will that be difficult for your family?

When accompanying a dying loved one through the end of life, what might you say or do to encourage a lasting peace?

FAMILY CAREGIVING

The best we can hope for in preparing a loved one for a good death, if there is such a thing, is to strengthen whatever sense of control he or she can retain over this most personal of passages...The most emotionally wrenching task for each family member is to find one's own way to let go...We are the ones who must give up control...The most important medicine during this time is honest conversation, guided by professionals and spiritual support.

—GAIL SHEEHY, *PASSAGES IN CAREGIVING*

CAREGIVING CAN BE one of the most demanding and satisfying activities of a lifetime. As a nation, we place an immense responsibility of personal care on the shoulders of family, friends and loved ones. There are an estimated fifty million Americans taking care of loved ones at home without pay. If you or a loved one are homebound, you may qualify for Medicare's Home Health Benefit. You can explore this resource through a link in the closing chapter.

If you're the patient, it's okay to need and ask for help. Expressing sincere appreciation to your caregivers, whether family or professional, goes a long way. Many of us are unsure of how and when to ask for help. Needing help with any "activities of daily living" (ADLs) is a useful benchmark. They are bathing, dressing, eating, toileting (incontinence), and mobility / transferring. If any of these have become an issue, it's time to recruit help.

It's not unusual for caregivers, when providing for a loved one at home, to become afraid that they're not doing enough or become uncertain of what's taking place and what to do next. An important part of hospice care is normalizing what's taking place. Learning more about the normal process of dying will alleviate much of the fear. Hopefully, this kind of support and reassurance lies within these pages or is a phone call away—ideally to your hospice team, not 911. Even when things go as well as possible, caregiving is still a demanding labor of love.

If you're a caregiver, either by profession or by loving necessity, it is important to include yourself in that circle of care. What you're doing is hard work. Ask yourself what is required to make it sustainable. Rest and recovery are essential. Also, talking with other caregivers is a helpful coping strategy.

A closing note: When a loved one or patient dies

after a long illness and the role of caregiver ends, there will likely be a vacuum and a full spectrum of related feelings of loss. Please know that this is normal and calls for generous selfcare. A diamond in the rough: Most every hospice agency offers bereavement resources to surviving family members.

HOSPICE (PART TWO)

LEE WAS WELL SUITED for hospice care. He made the team's job seem easy. He asked good questions, listened well, and communicated kindly and clearly. He embodied "the golden rule" and received loving respect in return. Lee died the way he lived. His final chapters reflected the same values that he taught his students and that he lived by. He chose peace in the end, and by virtue of his choices, he crafted an end-of-life scenario that he could manage and that his family could look back on with satisfaction. What I'll remember about Lee and am working to emulate is how he embodied holistic well-being, even in his dying time.

In the last twenty years, hospice agencies have evolved from being altruistic, independently owned non-profits to become mainstream participants in our national healthcare system. Hospice care is now available coast to coast in most every hospital, continuing care facility, and private home. Its availability waits on our willingness to accept that a cure is no longer possible and that further treatments may further compromise whatever quality of life remains.

Most people wait long into their illness to learn about hospice and to accept what it has to offer. Nearly thirty percent of hospice patients are referred in their last week of life, severely limiting the benefit to both patient and family.[1] A simple explanation: to receive Medicare's hospice benefit, a patient is normally required to discontinue life-prolonging treatments such as chemotherapy, radiation, ICU admission, surgery, and feeding tubes. You may recognize this as a grave disincentive that many clinicians believe needs to be addressed through updated Medicare legislation.

Even with forethought and planning, to finally accept that life is coming to an end is hard work. When given the opportunity to discuss a patient's hopes and fears, the hospice team is highly skilled at helping patients understand various care options that might be well-aligned with the patient's values and concerns.

Learning what hospice has to offer and saying "yes" to its model of care is not likely to shorten your life. Extensive research and supporting data show just the opposite. The implementation of early palliative care leading to the acceptance of hospice care not only leads to less suffering and more comfort, but longer life. It's counter-intuitive but a fact. No matter the setting, personalized, attentive care focused on quality of life is the best medicine.

The heart of hospice care is reclaiming the end of life as an essential human experience instead of a continuing medical battle. Hospice care is designed to acknowledge and support all aspects of a person: physical, emotional, mental, and spiritual. This is holistic medicine at its finest. Like palliative care, Hospice is provided by an interdisciplinary team, including a doctor, nurse, social worker, home health aide, and chaplain, as needed or requested.

Hospice has shown me time and again that with skillful pain management, dying can be acceptable, even peaceful. Ideally, hospice care gives a patient time to decide what a "good death" might look like and then to rally the loving support of family, friends, and a dedicated care team.

LOVE DISPELS FEAR

IN ATTENDING TO SUFFERING, the strongest medicine I know is love. The love that "bears all things, believes all things, hopes all things, and endures all things."[2] Its antithesis is fear. It's extremely difficult for the two to coexist—some say impossible. We each must choose time and again which to align with and to nurture. It's only natural to fear the end of life and the great unknown. It's in us. So is love if we choose to call on it. How does one do that? Perhaps by remembering a loved one's unconditional acceptance, or by saying a short prayer. I find love in stillness and through listening for the "quiet voice within." Like facing the sun, love's warmth can dispel fear and alleviate suffering every time we remember to turn toward it. Words fall short of capturing love's power to comfort, transform, and heal.

ADDITIONAL TOOLS

People are like stained glass windows. They sparkle and shine when the sun is out, but when the darkness sets in, their true beauty is revealed only if there is a light from within.

—Elizabeth Kubler-Ross

As a caregiver or patient, it's helpful to recognize and be familiar with Kubler-Ross's phases of grief. They are Denial, Anger, Bargaining, Depression, and Acceptance. (See Appendices for Link)

We're likely to cycle through these phases many times.

Denial is a useful coping strategy, at least for a time.

Remember to take breaks, even short ones to shift focus and attention.

Breathe deeply.... Exhaling fully.

Find something or someone to be grateful for. It's a remarkable antidote to what ails us.

Pray.... Have a conversation with the Power that is both beyond and within us.

Love.... Particularly that which appears unlovable—in the world around us and within our tender hearts.

Practice acceptance.... Love's first cousin.

Express creativity. Even if it's just to daydream or to imagine.

Find and use good humor as if it were medicine. It is.

Meditate for short periods of time, either sitting or walking...even lying down.

Use your imagination to visualize, remember, and cherish your favorite people, places, and the seminal moments of a lifetime. The more vivid you can make it by incorporating various senses—colors, sounds, smells, touch—the more benefit to your whole being.

Forgive others and ourselves. However old or tight the knot, let it loosen while there's still time.

PRACTICE SESSION:

PICK AN ACTIVITY from the list above and give yourself five to ten minutes each morning for a week to see how it feels. Explore the difference between thinking about forgiveness, for example, and allowing the truth of this healing balm to soften your heart and mind. What does it feel like to experience forgiveness? Consider selecting another activity the following week and doing the same.

Chapter Six

One Bright Morning, Gonna Fly Away Home

Sandy's renowned brain surgeon at UCSF Medical Center met with me briefly after her eight-hour operation. He appeared tired and had a right to be. He had successfully removed all he could of a spidery glioblastoma while preserving my ex-wife's ability to walk and talk, at least for now.

Without my having to ask, he said, "David, this will give her about eighteen months."

I swallowed hard and struggled to find the words to thank him. We shook hands and he turned to go.

"She'll be out of recovery in about an hour, and you can see her," he said, turning back.

I wandered outside the hospital, dazed, and found a nearby place to get a bowl of soup. Sitting in a quiet corner, I imagined how the next year or so might go. When the waitress delivered the check, it came with a handwritten note that said, "I'm sorry. I hope things get better." I hadn't said anything about the hospital. We hadn't even talked. As I left, I thanked her for her kindness.

Two weeks after surgery, prior to beginning radiation, with no hair and a handmade wool hat to cover the startling line of sutures around her skull, Sandy announced, "This will be the best year of my life!" That's how she was. A few weeks later, she headed off with friends to hike in Yosemite, while I stayed with our son Freeman. He shared his mother's optimism, and it wasn't for me, at least yet, to take his hopes away.

The differences between Sandy and me that once seemed insurmountable melted away in the face of her prognosis. She needed me and I needed to be there. It did turn out to be a remarkable year of seizing each day, one after another. I remember our last Christmas together and driving to a local nursery to find a live tree. We had loved our visits to the giant redwoods over the years, so when the owner suggested a baby sequoia, we brought it home to the living room and decorated it to the hilt.

Sandy was a force to be reckoned with. She had fifteen good months before the tumor regrew. The next three months were terrible for those of us who loved her. Yet, strangely enough, the truth of what was unfolding did not seem available to Sandy. We all knew the score, except for her. It was surreal. She wasn't in denial, per se, but she displayed a lack of capacity to grasp what was so evident to the rest of us. And that's how it went until the end.

Like an embryo, terminal cancer begins in a single cell. It replicates and grows, undetectably small for a time, then becomes apparent and runs its malicious course. Finally, the body has no more room to spare, and the life force surrenders. As her vital brain functions succumbed in the final months, adult capabilities gave way to childlike simplicity. Ultimately, Sandy returned to an infancy, no longer walking, or speaking, no longer reasoning—simply being. Her wide eyes were like windows, open to the beyond.

Sandy's choice to die at home allowed us significant freedom in contrast to a hospital setting. This autonomy gave us a precious measure of control and privacy. The pace was hers to set, the caregivers ours to choose. Each stage and process appeared to unfold naturally, as opposed to being treated as a medical procedure. The care and guidance from our local hospice was invaluable.

One Friday, eighteen months after life-saving surgery, Sandy's breathing turned rapid and shallow. Death was at our door patiently waiting its due and the door was open. Freeman was at school, which seemed like the right place for him. I sat at bedside, quietly reading aloud from Kahlil Gibran's *The Prophet*, one of Sandy's favorites. Our sister-in-law, Aleen, sat at the foot of the bed in prayer. An intravenous pump of morphine confined Sandy's pain to a remote corner of her being, allowing a tranquil spaciousness, albeit grievous, to fill the room.

As death stepped forward, Sandy's breathing bore an uncanny resemblance to when she gave birth. On both occasions, her personality was usurped by a more compelling force. Each time I felt that we were on hallowed ground. Each time came the awe of witnessing one of life's most powerful and mysterious passages. It felt comforting to continue to read to her, now from Gibran's chapter "On Death": "And what is it to cease breathing, but to free the breath from its restless tides, that it may rise and expand and seek God unencumbered?"

The intervals between breaths lengthened. They were now just small sips of air. I kept reading aloud, now from the closing chapter, "The Farewell": "And you shall see. And you shall hear... For in that day, you shall know the hidden purposes of all things, and you shall bless darkness as you bless light... Patient, over patient, is the captain of my ship. The wind blows, and restless are the sails; even the rudder begs direction; yet quietly my captain awaits my silence... I am ready. The stream has reached the sea, and once more the great mother holds her daughter against her breast." And with those very words, I looked up to see Sandy take her last breath.

In the stillness, Aleen and I listened, spellbound, to the audible sound of wings flapping as Sandy's spirit took flight. I can still hear them in my inner ear.

Eventually, the front door opened. Freeman called "I'm home!" and set his heavy backpack down. He walked in quietly and stopped near the door. He knew in a moment that his mother was gone. Sandy's head was propped up with an extra pillow. Freeman came closer and tentatively touched her skin.

"She feels cold," he said. "But it looks like she's smiling. She's not hurting anymore, is she?"

"It's true," Aleen answered.

"Dad, my friends walked home with me from school. Can I go out and play?" We held each other tightly for a moment, but I knew he needed to go. He went out and played with his friends for what felt like hours.

Aleen and I reverently cleaned and dressed Sandy's body and prepared for the undertaker to arrive.

A week or so later, on Easter Sunday, family and friends gathered in a local wooded park to celebrate Sandy's life and to say goodbye. Perhaps you've already imagined what became of the baby sequoia. With a portion of Sandy's cremains at its roots, a towering redwood stands there as a sentinel to this day.

FOR FURTHER CONVERSATION:

ONE OF THE HARDEST PARTS of life is seeing a loved one suffer. When that person is no longer suffering, even when death is the outcome, it's natural to feel relief amidst the grief. Have you experienced a version of this?

If your spouse or partner is still alive, would you be willing to talk with them about your hopes and fears around the end of life?

CONVERSATIONS WITH ONESELF

THERE ARE TIMES WHEN the best person to talk with is the one in the mirror. On a deep level, even in the face of great uncertainty, I believe that we can intuit exactly what we're up against. If we're willing to be honest with ourselves and to ask for guidance, then our innate wisdom can point the way. With patience and compassion, the practice of self-reflection can be both liberating and empowering. A footnote: If at first your inner critic shows up, ask instead to speak with your better angels.

Another way to approach the truth that lies beneath is to journal. As Sandy recovered from life-saving surgery, she began to write again. Over the next fifteen months she found great comfort in reflecting on her life and used her writing as a therapeutic tool for self-discovery. The process allowed her to search for and find meaning while inching toward acceptance. Even as the tumor regrew, bringing severe headaches, when asked how she was, Sandy would smile and say "fine." She meant it. As her personality succumbed, her spirit expressed itself with a clarity that defies description. For me, and others in her inner circle, she became a shining presence, a channel of innocence and a window of light.

If you're familiar with journaling, Sandy's experience likely makes sense to you. If you're not familiar with the practice, I encourage you to experiment. One key is to remember that the writing is for your eyes only. A popular exercise to bypass the mind's normal "editor" is to commit to a series of ten-minute writing sessions, each without stopping. Just keep the pen (or keys) moving for ten minutes. It doesn't have to look good, sound good, or even make sense. It's a way to access deeper layers of both personal and universal truth. Give it a try and see what comes up.

DYING AT HOME VERSUS AT THE HOSPITAL

WHEN ASKED ABOUT THEIR END-OF-LIFE WISHES, most people prefer to die at home and to avoid invasive measures. Yet currently two out of three deaths in the U.S. occur in institutional settings. One in three dies after a stay in the intensive care unit in the last three months of life.[1] When we're healthy, it's normal to idealize the notion of being kept comfortable at home. When we're terribly sick, receiving intravenous medications and needing help breathing, the hospital is a safer bet. A lot depends on the trajectory of one's disease. As for caregivers, most of us underestimate the demands of providing quality care at the end of life. Yet it stands out as one of the most profound and formative experiences of my life. It's also normal to overestimate the number of caregiving hours that hospice or home health can provide. "It takes a village" to die at home. This requires foresight and teamwork.

Regarding ethnic and cultural diversity, those who are able die at home, surrounded by family and friends, will benefit more fully from their cultural heritage and traditions. Unfortunately, at the hospital and nursing home, that opportunity is by and large surrendered.

HOSPICE (PART 3)

No matter the setting, unmanaged pain and agitation are the most common obstacles to a peaceful death. Hospice care is nationally recognized for skillful pain management. Morphine, when prescribed and administered by a hospice nurse, can be a godsend. It is commonly used at the end of life to quell pain and to relieve shortness of breath. Patients and family members sometimes worry that morphine will speed up the dying process, but there's no evidence to support this concern. In fact, the relief patients receive from morphine may allow then to live slightly longer.[2] When a patient is receiving morphine in the final hours, there will always be a last dose prior to death. It's not surprising for a family member to wonder if that dose was the cause of death. Not likely. It was just the final medication given prior to death's arrival.

Hospice care will soon mark its fiftieth anniversary in the United States. Most every boomer is generally familiar with hospice, and millions of us have a more personal connection. The hospice model is ideally suited to this generation's penchant for autonomy and control. Yet most patients still wait too long to say "yes" to what hospice has to offer. For lack of clear conversation with their doctors, many patients aren't aware that they're nearing the end of life. As a result, they may overuse life-prolonging treatment and underuse services that support quality of life and their goals of care.

Examples of life-prolonging treatment include chemotherapy, radiation, late-stage hospitalization, ICU admission, late-stage surgery, feeding tubes and MRIs. Each of the above tends to delay or exclude conversations about quality of life and what matters most to you. The result: a truncated hospice stay, if at all, and less focus on psychosocial, spiritual, and family support.

When it comes to the end of life, peace and quiet are important. Home hospice tends to be a much quieter experience than being in either a hospital or a nursing home. For most patients, let alone family members, this quality alone can make a huge difference. It can be one of the most important contributors to an acceptable death. Imagine the difference between an environment you and your family have some say over and the normal chaos of a busy hospital or nursing home unit. More hospitals and care homes are creating quieter places to die, but private space and control over the setting are limited. At its best, hospice is not a place as much as a way of seeing and valuing life that supports and champions a self-directed end.

SPIRITUAL CARE

If we fail to look at the emotional, psychological, and spiritual components at end of life, then we've truly missed the boat on providing whole person care.

—Dr. Patrice Richardson

Cicely Saunders's original model of hospice care addressed her patients' "total pain," which included emotional and existential distress. Spiritual care was an integral component of the holistic support Dr. Saunders and her team provided, and has remained a foundational part of hospice and palliative care to this day. Spiritual care is the heart of a chaplain's calling, and invites attention to one's faith, however it might be experienced.

Typically, when a chaplain first responds to a palliative or hospice referral, a spiritual assessment is in order. Usually this takes place quite informally during conversation. This approach is designed to identify how the patient describes their faith, or lack thereof, and to begin to understand how the patient is coping with their illness. In this context, religious beliefs and native spirituality are viewed as tools that can ease fear and discomfort, while fostering connection and peace of mind.

Faith, religion, and spirituality refer to the ways we seek and find meaning and purpose in our lives. It's the way we deepen our connection to the moment, to others, to nature, and to the Sacred, however we define it.[3] Over the course of a lifetime, most of us experience an ebb and flow in our faith and spirituality. As the end of life approaches—or perhaps more accurately, as we come to face and accept our mortality—faith often takes on a deeper importance. Whether one's faith is expressed outwardly in a religious manner or as a quiet, inward spirituality becomes uniquely personal.

From what I've seen at well over 10,000 bedsides, those who experience and allow themselves to rest in their faith are calmer, more accepting, and even expectant of what's to come. As a spiritual care provider, it's a privilege to be welcomed into the room, to offer a calm presence, and to accompany a fellow traveler through some of life's most difficult terrain. Spiritual care isn't too complicated. Please remember that with clear intent, anyone can muster the tools of listening from the heart, providing undivided attention, and offering the gift of quiet companionship.

PEEKING THROUGH THE VEIL

FOR AT LEAST 2,500 YEARS, religious teachers, prophets, and mystics have spoken about a veil between the world of the living and the dead. It's said that the veil is particularly thin as death approaches. While words can point to it, experiencing it is another matter, and one not easily forgotten. Many of us have already brushed against it. Some, by being at the bedside of a dying loved one. Others through a dedicated yoga or breathing practice. Some through deep and prolonged meditation.

Others through devote prayer or chanting. In addition, the boomers have other guides to thank.

With Aldous Huxley's account of his experiences with mescaline, *The Doors of Perception*, and the widespread use of hallucinogens in the 1960s and 70s, the boomers have been busy exploring the outer (and inner) reaches of consciousness. In 2013, the National Institute of Health reported that an estimated 32 million adult Americans have used either mescaline, peyote, psilocybin ("magic mushrooms"), or LSD.[4]

When the federal government outlawed these hallucinogens in 1970, they went "underground," yet they have continued to be available both for recreational and therapeutic use. Over the years, a growing number of intrepid researchers and psychologists have insisted that these hallucinogens allow the user to overcome the mortal fear of death, often with a transcendent, lasting effect. Thanks to celebrated author Michael Pollan's in- depth study, *How to Change Your Mind*, mescaline and its first cousin, psilocybin, are once again topics of mainstream conversation. Why now? In part, because a new generation is moving into position to question how we die and is suggesting a better way with less fear and more awareness.

To help connect the dots, it was Elizabeth Kubler-Ross who invited the relatively unknown meditation teacher, Stephen Levine, to join her workshops on death and dying in the 1970s. Levine went on to write his bestseller, *Who Dies? An Investigation of Conscious Living and Conscious Dying,* which points beyond the veil and has endeared him to many. A memorable aspect of Levine's later workshops was his standing invitation to attendees who had had a near-death experience, to address the group. Invariably, humble, and ordinary people would recount having been pronounced dead, only to be resuscitated and regain their faculties. With few exceptions, these people did not "peek" through the veil, but stepped through to the other side. Their accounts are remarkably consistent. What they experienced when separated by "death" from their bodies was profound. As near as words can describe, they experienced peace, beauty, and light. Most relevant here, they reported that their fear of death had vanished and not returned.

By acknowledging and sitting with our fear of death—by not running for cover—we each have an opportunity to understand and transform ourselves at the deepest level. To bear witness to another's dying time, or to anticipate our own, can be to stand in wonder, not knowing, in awe of life's greatest mystery. As you've already glimpsed, this has the power to not only transform how we die, but—perhaps more importantly—to transform how we live.

For Further Conversation:

WHETHER YOU'RE A RELIGIOUS or secular person, please ask yourself, what are my core beliefs? What do I hold to be true? Which of these truths will serve me right now and as life presents its closing chapters? What do I need to remember? To invite? To deepen? And to savor? Our saving grace, whatever it might be, waits on our welcome.

Practice Session:

FOR MANY OF US, going to church is no longer attractive or practical. Yet there may still be a "house of worship" somewhere inside us. Visualize or imagine, if you will, your old connection to church, synagogue, mosque, or the great outdoors, coming alive again in your mind's eye. Close your eyes, breathe deeply, and let yourself be transported there. Allow your senses to rekindle and fully experience this place again. Picture brilliant light, or sacred darkness, enveloping you. Are there comforting sounds or smells? What feels most alive within you? Offer whatever prayers might come to you, allowing the peace of this place to wash over you. Imagine kneeling or bowing in gratitude, giving thanks for the comfort and refuge this place still offers you.

Assisted Living

Chapter Seven

Still Here

THERE ARE TIMES WHEN DYING goes as smoothly as one could hope. It was this way for my friend, Margie. She would be delighted to know that her story was being told.

I met Margie late in her life through a family friendship. She had the good fortune, through inheritance, to afford living in an exclusive continuing care community on the Mainline outside Philadelphia. Margie and her husband had joined the community many years earlier and lived there independently. As they aged and downsized, they moved into a comfortable apartment in the community's personal care wing. They were surrounded by engaging neighbors and enjoyed sharing their meals in a lovely community dining room. There was a complete health clinic on the premises with 24-hour nursing care available as needed—as eventually it was—for each resident aging in place.

During one of our lunchtime visits, Margie

asked me to reach an old book from atop her library shelf. Her modest collection reflected a lifelong love of reading, both fiction and non-fiction. You can tell a lot about a person by the books he or she keeps. Margie loved history, art, music, and travel. But this book's importance was that it held a faded article she wanted me to see, clipped long ago and tucked away for later reference. The writer conveyed a quiet "secret" she'd discovered, a long-practiced custom that had been entrusted to her by word of mouth. The writer's pearl: that we could choose the time of our death by giving up eating and drinking.

With an inquisitive lift of her eyebrows, Margie asked me, "Have you ever heard of such a thing?"

I smiled in reply. "Yes, it's how my mother chose to go."

Margie's face softened, reflecting calm reassurance. Her gaze was down and forward, and she nodded slowly to herself. These pivotal conversations need not be long. The mission is to convey what's most important to a person. A simple understanding between us was sealed.

Now into her early 90s, with her husband long passed, Margie's bus trips with her fellow residents to hear the Philadelphia Orchestra had dwindled. As with many seniors, incontinence can be a determining factor in how far afield one travels. Her beloved children continued to visit and give her cause to soldier on, but it was plain to see that she was in decline. Although the staff helped her with activities of daily living (ADLs) in the apartment, Margie's instinct was to downsize and simplify by transitioning to the assisted living wing. Accompanied by favorite family photographs, a comfortable chair for visitors, and an African Violet or two, Margie moved into a single room with a picture window. Her medical team was now at her beck and call, just steps away.

What made all the difference was neither her good fortune nor her manageable decline, but her graceful acceptance combined with clear, direct communication. Having an exit strategy that matched her values brought peace of mind. Margie confided in her doctors her intent to die on her own terms and in her own time. They, in turn, entrusted her with an honest prognosis and pledged their support. She and her family spoke comfortably about important choices that lay ahead while embracing the present. There were no secrets, and little was left unspoken. It was an honor to be included as her chaplain.

Family and friends came and went from her small room. Her son installed a bird feeder outside the picture window that became a flutter of activity. Margie continued to read and to ready herself. When one daughter was reluctant to offer her blessing, Margie was gently resolute. As often happens, her body was requiring less food, and her appetite conspired to support her plan, until one day she stopped eating. A few days later, her need to use the toilet diminished, and she let us know that "the day" had arrived. She toasted to our health, thanked us one and all for our loving support, and had her last glass of water.

Margie was alert and expectant for the next few

days. When her mouth became dry, her nurse would gently moisten Margie's lips and mouth. The hospice team was fully on board, and they prescribed Ativan for Margie's low-level anxiety, as well as maintenance doses of morphine to quell her underlying pain and relax her breathing. She was resting when I visited to say goodbye, but she woke easily and opened her eyes.

Clearing her throat, with a wry smile, she managed to say: "I'm still here," evidently a bit perplexed as to why.

I read in her eyes the question *How much longer?* and attempted to reassure her with a gentle touch, saying, "All in good time." The next day, her eyes closed, and she dropped beneath the surface, not to return. Her loved ones began a bedside vigil, as old as time.

A day later, in the dead of night, our beloved Margie slipped away.

Is there a chance that our end-of-life decisions are made years in advance? Do we make them ourselves, or are they determined by happenstance and factors beyond our control—for example, by our family of origin, our health, or our self-care (or lack thereof)? How do we reach our most important decisions? Do we come to them alone or in concert with others? I think we each must decide upon them ourselves, with foresight as well as a willingness to pivot as new circumstances present themselves.

THOUGH MARGIE WAS OF THE SILENT GENERATION, her self-determination and confident communication with her family and clinicians models the themes that baby boomers are choosing to emulate. What speaks to you about Margie's character?

Margie's clear-eyed vision, seeded by an Ann Lander's column years earlier, set a direction for her family and care team to follow. What's alive and growing within you that could well blossom in the final chapters?

LONGEVITY VERSUS QUALITY OF LIFE

We are the beneficiaries and victims of scientific success. Serious, chronic illness is an invention of the late 20th century, the fruit of our species' intellectual prowess, the culmination of scientific progress.

—DR. IRA BYOCK, *THE BEST CARE POSSIBLE*

DR. IRA BYOCK HAS BEEN A GUIDING force in the palliative care movement over the past forty years, and I want to acknowledge his significant contributions as a gifted clinician, educator, author, and activist.

Through medicine and life-saving technology, the silent generation and now the boomers live an average of twenty-five years longer than their parents.[1] This longevity is an unprecedented achievement. As eight out of ten of us now die gradually, we have the novel opportunity to have a voice in how, where, and when we die. Although people are learning to be proactive, many are quietly suffering slow and tragic deaths.

Our nation's 15,000 Skilled Nursing Facilities, with 1.7 million licensed beds, are overflowing.[2] An estimated 6.2 million Americans over the age of sixty-five are living with Alzheimer's Disease. One out of three Americans over the age of eighty-five are afflicted with the disease.[3] Our thirst for longevity combined with no exit strategy has created a tremendous burden. You can see it in any hospital, skilled nursing facility, and in most every family. Few experiences bring this reality home quicker than caring for an aging and dependent loved one. What can we do to alleviate the situation?

Each of us can be clearer and more outspoken about what we want AND what we don't want in preparation for and during our dying time. If our goal is to live as long as possible, it's important to say so. The hospital team will oblige. If living as well as possible is our goal, it's important to make that clear. That way, our loved ones and clinical team can help us weigh the benefits of various treatments alongside their burdens and risks of ill effects.

Technology can keep a patient "alive" almost indefinitely. In too many cases the prescribed use of life support has outstripped morals and ethics. When is it morally and ethically acceptable to allow for death? This is a deeply personal question that begs thoughtful reflection and response. If this question is not addressed, the institutional default is well established and will be the default course of action. You can count on it. Many procedures and treatments keep a person alive even when there is no chance that they will improve or leave the hospital. Prolonged misery and moral distress are too often the outcome.

BIOETHICS

ORIGINALLY A RESPONSE TO UNETHICAL RESEARCH by physicians during wartime, the field of bioethics has evolved to guide and protect both patients and clinicians in making difficult decisions. Hospital ethics committees have become the field's most visible arbiter. The dilemmas they address often pertain to end-of-life decision-making, specifically the decision of whether to continue, refuse, or withdraw from life-saving measures.

It was the Patient Self-Determination Act that formalized patients' right to refuse life-sustaining medical treatment, which was when the advance directive came into general use. Today, bioethics are as relevant as ever due to the growing emphasis on shared decision-making and patient and family-centered care. In the event of an entrenched disagreement regarding patient care, whether family or clinician-centered, an ethics review can be requested.

THE CONTINUING CARE
COMMUNITY

THE CONTINUING CARE COMMUNITY (CCC) is a popular model for those who wish to age in place, and who have the financial resources to afford it. This senior living concept has been honed and improved over the years. My favorite rendition, grounded in old school Quaker values, is the Kendal Senior Living Communities (see Kendal.org). The peace of mind and relative security of living in a community where an appropriate level of care can be easily adjusted as we age is an attractive investment.

But buyer beware: There are personal care homes that do NOT offer skilled nursing. A resident's increased need for nursing services can quickly lead to a "thirty-day notice" of discharge. The fine print in the welcome package (often a fifty-page document) will spell out the criteria for discharge. Be sure to take the necessary time to understand a prospective community's strengths and limitations.

DEMENTIA AND MEMORY CARE

MARGIE WAS FORTUNATE enough to be able to think clearly up until her dying day. For countless others, it's a different story. As we live longer, the odds increase that we will either be taking care of a loved one with dementia or that we will become the one requiring memory care. Over time, it's likely, we will be both—a very sobering prospect indeed. For me, this is one of the most compelling reasons to be proactive in planning ahead and in talking candidly with my son (my agent) about my values and preferences.

Advanced dementia ranks among the slowest and most insidious ways to die. Caring for a loved one with dementia can be a full-time job, often without pay, for years on end. On average, a person with Alzheimer's disease lives four to eight years after diagnosis. One in three seniors dies with Alzheimer's disease or some other form of dementia.[4] There is currently no cure, only medications that slow and draw out the dying time. While patients with advanced dementia may benefit from conversations intent on easing their suffering, after a certain point, such conversations appear to be of little benefit.

More staggering figures: There are currently over sixteen million Americans taking care of family members who are living with Alzheimer's. Approximately twenty-five percent of these caregivers (roughly four million) are "sandwich caregivers"— meaning they care simultaneously for an aging parent and for a child under age eighteen. Two-thirds of dementia caregivers are women. One out of three are older than 65.[5] Two-thirds of those who die of dementia will do so in nursing homes.[6] This flurry of numbers and information can be overwhelming.

It takes a coordinated, team effort to provide quality care, whether at the hospital, at a skilled nursing facility, or at home. Willingness to discuss this possible eventuality and include specific guidance in the advance directive can alleviate untold anguish.

One of the most heart-wrenching chores I've had while working in skilled nursing facilities is feeding pureed meals to non-verbal patients with advanced dementia. If I can no longer feed myself, I've asked my son to cease and desist. It's written into my advance directive, along the lines of Katy Butler's suggested wording near the end of chapter four. While there is no sure way to avoid ending up in a memory care unit, the best proactive hedge I'm aware of is to choose comfort measures only in one's advance directive, including the option of no antibiotics in the event of a nursing home placement. This leaves the door open for the old person's friend (pneumonia) to provide a merciful exit at some point.

ARTIFICIAL FEEDING

As we face serious, life-threatening conditions, it may become impossible to swallow normally or to take in enough food or water to survive. Both can be administered through tubes. Here's how it works. A thin tube, called an "NG tube," can be inserted through the nose, which descends through the back of the throat to the stomach. More invasively, a broader tube, called a "PEG tube," is surgically implanted through the abdomen into the stomach. Water and nutritional liquids can then be gently pumped through either of these tubes. This process works best if the patient needs a short time to recover from surgery or a sudden illness. Tube feeding, however, is highly controversial if the patient is chronically ill, or their vital organs have already begun to shut down.

Adverse side effects of artificial feeding may include aspiration and infection caused by undigested food coming back up into the lungs, or the systemic buildup of excess fluids—particularly in the lungs or stomach, if vital organs are already compromised. On occasion, the patient's hands may also need to be tied down so as not to pull out the tube(s).

If you, your doctor(s), or your agent decide to accept a feeding tube, it's important to discuss and to agree ahead of time how long a fair trial might be. What are the goals of care? What if your health gets worse or if you can't talk or think clearly? Note well: discontinuing artificial feeding can be more emotionally fraught than beginning it.

If you and your care team decide not to accept artificial feeding or to discontinue it, there are sound options to keep you as comfortable as possible. Make sure these options are part of the discussion from the start. Ask the doctor who knows you best to discuss the potential benefits and burdens and to help you decide. If you're inclined not to accept tube feeding, it's best to let your doctor and agent know ahead of time and to document it. When food and water are no longer able to be given or assimilated, you will die naturally from your underlying condition(s). Most patients report not feeling hungry. With a dry mouth, attentive oral care can make all the difference.

CONVERSATIONS BETWEEN FAMILY AND CLINICIANS

When a patient is unconscious or has lost the capacity to make rational decisions, the medical team will turn to the patient's healthcare agent or next of kin for guidance. A skilled clinician will ask important questions and listen well. The best-case scenario would be to anticipate such an occasion and to be prepared to speak for the patient to clearly relay their preferences. It's a given that we can't anticipate every twist and turn of a complicated illness. As agents, we just do our best to ask good questions, to collaborate with the medical team in making decisions, and to trust that we know our loved ones well enough to represent them as faithfully as we can.

With a deeper understanding established, the clinical team and family can make mutual decisions about how to proceed in a way that shares control and honors the patient's values. If this sounds like good palliative care practice, you're right.

If you had advanced dementia and could not speak or feed yourself, what would your wishes be?

If you could no longer feed yourself, but still had capacity, would you want to be spoon fed? Under what conditions would you want to be fed through a nose tube or a stomach tube? Under what conditions would you want all intake of food and liquid to be stopped, and allow you to be on your way?

Please discuss this with your agent and add these preferences to your advance directive.

Chapter Eight

Running Out of Options

Robert was thrown from his metal ladder as 60,000 volts of electricity surged through him. He had been asked to cover for the warehouse foreman that humid morning, and to reboot the plant's faulty electrical system. His heart likely stopped before he hit the ground, never to beat again. They reached his wife, Tasha, at home. She was stoic at first, numb and protected by shock. That would pass.

A week later, in mourning and now deep in grief, Tasha met with her doctor. He attempted to console her with the unexpected news that, at thirty-five years old, she was pregnant with her first child. Her shock only deepened, compounding a loss that would shadow her for life. Eight months later she gave birth to Trevor, a beautiful and energetic boy, born with developmental disabilities. He became the love of her life.

The arc of a lifetime defies simple description. It

was fifty years later when I met Tasha at Reading Hospital, after her nurse had suggested a pastoral visit. Tasha was eighty-five years old, feisty, and cantankerous, and spoke her mind. I liked her right away. Over the course of a few visits, at the hospital and at rehab, a bond developed between us. She asked for my help at a time when she "had no one." I told her that I would do my best.

Eventually Tasha was discharged home to her small third floor apartment in subsidized housing next to the oldest volunteer fire department in our country. It was rarely a quiet neighborhood. Tasha had rallied time and again, from heartbreak and widowhood to heart attack and resuscitation by CPR and a 500-volt defibrillator. She lived with renal failure and arthritic knees, which created wicked bone-on-bone pain. Between neighbors and good Samaritans, Tasha managed to cobble together one or two visits a week to a nearby dialysis clinic, which kept her alive.

One evening, exhausted from a day at the clinic, Tasha went to sit at her kitchen table, but misjudged the edge of her straight back chair. She landed on the bare floor and heard her hip crack beneath her. She screamed out, knowing immediately that her cherished independence had come to an end.

The fire department responded quickly and got her to the hospital. By the time she remembered my phone number, she had been x-rayed and was awaiting a verdict from the hip surgeon. When I reached her bedside, she was heavily medicated but awake enough to recognize me and to reach out her hand. The very motion shifted her position, and she cried out in pain. Her nurse came in quickly, and asked what had I done, to elicit a smile. Humor continues to be an effective medicine, but only surgery would stem Tasha's internal bleeding at the hip and assuage the knifing pain.

Physically and emotionally broken, and unable to find a comfortable position, Tasha was furious with herself for having fallen. She directed her anger toward her caregivers. It wasn't pretty. She needed skillful pain management—which takes time to fine-tune. Hip surgery was postponed to allow for her next dialysis treatment, which only deepened her misery. There was no easy way out. As is so often the case with frail elders, her fall marked the beginning of Tasha's final chapter. Talking about her loss of mobility was upsetting, but it needed to happen.

Sitting at her bedside, a week after the operation, I asked, "How are you doing?"

She frowned and shook her head from side to side. She was still in considerable pain, more so from her arthritis than from her hip. In addition, she was suffering from a feeling of profound loss. The doctors were saying that rehab, if it was even possible, would take one to two months. "What do you think we should do?" she asked.

I paused a moment. "I'm afraid we're running out of options."

Her reply was honest and direct. "I may not be able to walk again. I think I need to let go of my apartment. Will you help me?"

"Of course. I'll do whatever I can."

And that was that. The next stop was a brief re-hab, which was called short because Tasha couldn't bear any weight. Despite her new hip, the trauma of her fall combined with the resulting entropy would not allow her to walk again. A Hoyer lift was used to transfer her to a wheelchair to get her to dial-ysis. After a few months, there were days she just couldn't stand the pain and refused to get out of bed. She called me to talk.

"I think I'm ready to throw in the towel. Is that wrong?" she asked.

"No, it's not wrong. When I put myself in your place, I think I'd feel the same way."

There was a long pause before she spoke again. "If I stop dialysis, how long do you think I'll have?"

"Normally, just a couple weeks." I paused, want-ing to give her time to respond. She was quiet. "Ta-sha, tell me what's most important to you."

"To see my son again. To not be in pain. To not have to struggle anymore." Through her tears her voice was clear and unwavering. I could tell that she still had capacity and that she'd had enough.

The next two weeks went quickly. One morning, Trevor was brought from his group home about an hour away to the nursing home. I met him there and walked him to his mother's room. He had gotten a fresh haircut and was neatly dressed, wearing new sneakers that his mother had ordered for him. He appeared anxious, and no wonder. There were many disturbing sights, sounds and smells. It was a heart wrenching visit for them both. He was silent most of the time, looking down at the floor.

At one point he asked, "Mom where will you be buried?"

"Next to your father," she said.

"Will I be there someday, too?"

She nodded yes and reached out for him. He gently held her while they cried in each other's arms.

She reached to her bedside table and offered Trevor an envelope. "Here," she said, "I want you to have some spending money."

He opened it carefully. As he counted out fifty dollars, he came alive again, thinking of all he could buy on his way home. "Thanks, Mom...I better go now." And he gave her a quick parting hug. That was the last time they saw each other.

I visited her as often as I could between shifts at the hospital. We talked quietly and I encouraged her to reminisce, particularly about the gift of the past twenty-one years since her heart attack. Over the next few days, as the toxins built up in her body, she became weaker, grew weary, and slept more, until the day came when she didn't wake up. Her breathing was slow and calm, and she appeared to be at peace. Trevor chose not to come, saying that he wanted to remember her when she was awake. When I saw him next, it was to join me in burying Tasha's cremains in their small family plot.

DESPITE OUR UNIQUENESS, our health trajectories fit familiar patterns. Tasha's end-stage renal disease combined with a broken hip in her mid-eighties led to a predictable end. If you're living with chronic or life-threatening illness, such as chronic obstructive pulmonary disease (COPD) or heart disease, are you aware of how your illness normally progresses? If not, what hard questions could you bring to your doctor(s) to plan accordingly? For example: "Doctor, please be honest with me. What's my best-case scenario in the year ahead? And what's the worst?"

911

TASHA OWES HER LATER LIFE TO A TEAM of first responders. A quick arrival, electric paddles, and cardiopulmonary resuscitation (CPR) brought Tasha back to life and gave her an additional twenty-one years to live. When our national 911 system began in 1968, the only emergency medical technicians (EMTs) who made house calls were firemen or the hospital ambulance team. If a person was unfortunate enough to have a heart attack or stroke at home, it was usually catastrophic. Today there are nearly 300,000 EMTs and an additional 100,000 paramedics registered across the United States. This legion of first responders has not only changed the delivery of healthcare but also increased our life expectancy.

An estimated 240 million calls are made to 911 in the United States each year. In many areas, eighty percent or more are from wireless devices. Today's standard response time for ninety percent of all life-threatening incidents is five minutes.[1] This helps explain why today relatively few people still die of heart attacks.

When the EMTs arrive on the scene, they are legally and honor-bound to attempt resuscitation and provide life support. The notable exception: when there is a "POLST" document or an "out-of-hospital DNR" prominently displayed or immediately available. For lack of this, many terminally ill patients end up in the emergency department on life support, even though they had an advance directive instructing otherwise.

PHYSICIAN'S ORDERS FOR LIFE SUSTAINING TREATMENT (POLST)

IF YOUR ADVANCE DIRECTIVE is sitting in a drawer at home, as thorough and well-crafted as it may be, it WILL NOT be effective in an urgent situation. Many clinicians view the Physician's Orders for Life Sustaining Treatment form (POLST) as an essential and more useful tool to minimize undue suffering. Note well: a hard copy is intended to travel with us from one care setting to the next, in addition to being scanned into our medical record.

Ask your primary care doctor or attending physician at the hospital if completing a POLST form would be appropriate. To emergency responders and hospital clinicians, it's the most recognizable, efficient, and effective way to communicate one's treatment preferences. It's standard practice to print it on bright pink paper. First responders are bound by law to resuscitate unless a POLST or DNR form is in clear sight. Best practice: Tape a bright copy to your refrigerator or bedroom wall.

CARDIO-PULMONARY RESUSCITATION (CPR)

CPR DOESN'T WORK AS WELL as Hollywood would have us believe. It works best if you're healthy with no underlying illness, and best if it can be given within minutes of when your heart or breathing stops. CPR does not work well if you're older and weak, if you have chronic health problems, or if you have an illness that can no longer be treated.

CPR includes giving quick chest compressions, strong enough to break ribs, for as long as needed until a pulse has been re-established, or until the patient is declared dead. In a hospital setting, CPR can be administered on and off for up to an hour. The resuscitation efforts can also include mechanical assistance with breathing, as well as electrical shocks and medications, called "pressors," all to restart the heart and lungs.

If our heartbeat or breathing stops, CPR may or may not work. If you're in the hospital and get CPR, you have a one in five chance of it working and leaving the hospital alive. This includes all age groups. If you're older and weaker, whether at the hospital or from a skilled nursing facility, there is a two to three percent chance that CPR will restart your heart and lungs and that you will leave the facility alive.[2]

The time to decide if you want CPR is when you're well and have the facts you need to make an informed decision. Ask questions and talk to your doctor(s) and loved ones. If you want CPR, it would be good to understand what results you could expect given your age and condition. What would your goals be? What quality of life would be acceptable? Or unacceptable? If you don't want CPR, you need to tell your doctor and your family and have it documented.

What would lead me to have my agent decline CPR? Some examples: if I could no longer breathe without a machine; if I could no longer think or talk; or if I could no longer recognize my loved ones.

DIALYSIS

TASHA WAS ONE OF APPROXIMATELY 700,000 patients in the U.S. being kept alive at any given time by hemodialysis. This four-hour treatment, often provided three times a week, removes toxins from the body when the kidneys are no longer able. Many patients have been receiving the treatments for years. For most, if they were to stop, death would come quickly, usually in a couple of weeks. Many patients have a love/hate relationship with their complete dependence on this technology. In a large survey of patients receiving dialysis to support chronic kidney disease, sixty-one percent reported that they regretted initiating dialysis, and fifty-two percent reported that they chose dialysis because a physician told them it was the only way to stay alive.[3] There are rich and controversial incentives for the medical community to initiate and perpetuate dialysis treatments. It's a HUGE business. Two companies, DaVita and Fresenius, control roughly eighty percent of the U.S. market, valued at $24.7 billion annually. For reference, there are more dialysis centers in the United States than there are Burger King Restaurants.[4]

PREVENTING TRAUMATIC FALLS
(DOWN STEPS, OFF CURBS, OVER PETS, AND JUST GOING TO THE BATHROOM)

MOST FRAIL SENIORS FEAR FALLING above all else, and for good reason. Across the United States, every nineteen minutes an aging adult dies from a fall, often from a traumatic brain bleed and a protracted stay in the ICU. Every eleven seconds, an aging adult is treated in an emergency department for a fall.[5]

As with Tasha, one misstep can drastically change an elderly person's life. Most seniors never regain the level of mobility, function, and confidence they enjoyed prior to a serious fall. In an extensive study, only one in five seniors were able to live independently after being hospitalized from a fall.[6]

Many seniors, often due to vanity, are reluctant to use canes and walkers, even though these devices can play a vital role in staying safe. A little-known fact: Bifocals and progressive lens can distort people's vision and depth perception while they are looking down and walking, which can lead to a fall.

Accidents will happen, yet a few simple precautions may prevent an untimely fall and a world of trouble. "Fall-proof" the home. For the elderly, particularly when using a walker, a simple throw rug can become deadly. Firmly secure rugs to the floor or clear them out of the way. It's best to keep rooms free of clutter and electrical cords. Keep stairways well-lit and have sturdy handrails on both sides. In the bathroom, install grab bars beside the tub, shower, and toilet. Take a few minutes to reorganize kitchen and bedroom shelves to minimize the need to bend over or reach up to retrieve commonly used items. If dizziness or poor balance is a recurring problem, consider asking your doctor to review your medicines with an eye for adverse side effects.

PRACTICE SESSION:

PLEASE SLOW DOWN. Realize that EVERY step counts, and that it takes only one misstep to ruin a good life. If there are simple upgrades that can make your living space safer, ask for help in accomplishing them. As for the great outdoors, potential pitfalls may be no farther than a walk to the car or the mailbox.

SKILLED NURSING FACILITY (SNF)

Tasha was biding her time. Imaginary thinking provided her solace that she would someday walk again. In the meantime, she accepted the daily ordeal of Hoyer lifts and wheelchair transfers as a devil's bargain. During our daily phone conversations, she vented about the slow response to her "call bell" and her long wait between visits from aides. She had bedsores from not being moved enough, and a rash from sitting in wet and soiled briefs. The food wasn't very good, and her sleep was often interrupted by screams for help coming from the room next door. Unfortunately, none of this is unusual at the humble level of Medicare-funded Skilled Nursing. There are over one million Americans currently living under similar conditions.[7]

Too many people die in a way and in a place that is not of their choosing. One reason: a stubborn unwillingness to think about death, talk about it, or plan accordingly. Most people who find themselves in skilled nursing facilities swore they would never end up there. Another reason: People run out of better options. At one end of the continuum are those fortunate enough to afford a continuing care community that offers an in-house transition from independent living to assisted living, and finally to skilled nursing, which may include memory care. This graduated model tends to be the most expensive senior living option.

For those living on a modest fixed income, a shared room at a Medicare/Medicaid certified nursing home is a likely outcome. While most people would prefer to stay at home and age in place, diminished health and/or lack of an adequate support team often doesn't allow it. It then becomes time to investigate various assisted living options.

Practice Session:

HERE IS A BUDDHIST EQUANIMITY PRACTICE that can be useful during these times. Find a quiet and comfortable place for five to ten minutes. Take a few calming, centering breaths, and slowly recite and imagine the following:

"All things arise and pass away.

Joys, sorrows, events, and people, arise and pass away.

This is how it is right now.

May I be at peace with how it is right now.

May I find rest amidst the changes.

May I learn to see the arising and passing away

of all things with equanimity and balance.

May I be open, aware, and at peace.

All beings are heirs to their own actions.

Our joys and sorrows arise and pass away,

following the conditions and deeds created by us.
While I deeply love and care for others,
in the end, their happiness and suffering
depend on their thoughts and actions,
and not my wishes for them.
May I bring compassion and equanimity to my heart
and mind, and to the events of the world.
May I find balance and peace amidst it all."[8]

Chapter Nine

A Last Resort

The test of a civilization is how it cares for its helpless members.

—Pearl Buck, Nobel Laureate

Margie's plush 'retirement community' in Chapter Seven stands at one end of the long-term care continuum. Tasha's skilled nursing facility rests in the middle, with Medicaid-certified nursing homes holding down the other end. These Medicaid-certified facilities provide an essential service, yet are often considered a last resort, leading many of us to say, "Promise never to put me in a place like that." Just setting foot inside the front door can be heart-wrenching. The accompanying sights, sounds, and smells of housing our most vulnerable elders is disturbingly consistent from coast to coast. In case you haven't visited such a place, let me take you for a short tour. That said, since the ravages of the Covid-19 pandemic, a visit can't be assured.

Covid-19 took devastating advantage of the

close, communal contact which was considered normal at this modest level of care. While new precautions have been enacted, much is unchanged. As we leave the front desk, we're likely to encounter residents, often in their wheelchairs, lining the halls. Some hunger for contact and attention. Others are 'parked' near the nurses' station for closer supervision. Few seem to interact with each other, yet they relish the chance to meet a new person. Some will strike up a conversation, as if you're an old friend. Others may call out for a favor or ask a question out of left field. Coherent conversations are hard to come by. Residents will often be slouched over or asleep in their chairs, lost in a world of their own. It's also normal to find people clustered around a large TV, watching an old classic. Hearing cries for help or screaming in the distance is not uncommon.

Few family members have enough fortitude to visit regularly. Most residents, even those with serious cognitive disability, seem to know and feel when they've been abandoned. It's a shame. For aging Americans who have just been getting by or living below the poverty line for years, end of life can be more of the same, only worse. Spartan living quarters, filled with frail and disabled bodies, many of whom are suffering from advanced dementia, can be a harrowing environment. Consider that the average length of stay in assisted living is twenty-eight months. Add to the mix an average resident to staff ratio of fifteen to one, caregivers who are minimally paid and often underappreciated but are in truth the residents' guardian angels.

In sitting with nursing home residents, listening to various stories, I often find myself saying, "I wish things had turned out differently." The familiar response is "Me too," or perhaps just an outstretched hand in recognition that someone still cares. This is the dark side of a package deal handed to each of us through the extraordinary medical advances of the twentieth century.

The baby boom came in response to an intoxicating mix of post-war optimism and prosperity. It was easy to have more children and to believe that there would be a good life for all. For many it's held true. Yet death waits patiently its due, whether it be in Samarra, San Antonio, Los Angles, or New York. Now older and wiser, the boomers are uniquely suited to face and define their later lives and dying time. As more clinicians learn to meet the aging boomers where they are, and ask them what matters most, our healthcare industry will hopefully find incentives to serve the boomers' evolving needs, both as caregivers and ultimately, as patients.

FOR FURTHER CONVERSATION:

DO YOU KNOW AN ELDERLY PERSON who lives alone and can't get out easily? Would you be willing to call and offer to visit? Do you know anyone living at a nursing home? How would it be to drop by once a week for a half hour? In both cases, can you find the courage to ask about and quietly bear witness to their grief?

NEARING DEATH / THE VIGIL

I am of the nature to grow old. I am of the nature to be sick. I am of the nature to die. All that is dear to me and everyone I love are of the nature to change.

—Thich Nhat Hanh

Death is not extinguishing the light; it is only putting out the lamp because the dawn has come.

—Rabindranath Tagore

As Death Approaches, and the medical team musters the courage to tell us that there's no more that can be done to treat our illness, we must decide how best to cope. Please remember that we each have a profound say in how we live until we die. As a patient, no matter the setting, the time leading up to death can range from being a nightmare to being hallowed ground. Often it turns out to be both. As a caregiver, friend, or loved one, please take heart in knowing that your time and attention paid to the one dying is priceless, no matter how difficult the journey.

Dying is simultaneously a physical experience AND an emotional and spiritual event. Like a woman's labor in giving birth, the body's innate wisdom will do what it needs to complete the task at hand. Returning to Maslow's Hierarchy of Needs, as our physical needs are met, pain relief for example, our attention is then freed up to address emotional needs, for reassurance or forgiveness perhaps.

Realize that our final days and hours are affected by the emotional tenor of what takes place in the room. What's said or left unsaid? What is the tone of people's reminiscing and of the stories being told? What music or TV station is on? What prayers, if any are being offered? All of this contributes to how the dying time will go and what will be remembered.

When we accompany our loved ones and attend to their emotional needs, the door opens for the spiritual and sacred nature of dying to present itself. This can unfold quite naturally, and while it may be more challenging in a hospital or nursing home, it's doable. As a family member or friend, be clear in talking with clinicians about your hopes and intentions during this final chapter. Foster vigilance and a heightened awareness of what's unfolding, both spoken and silent; allowing for what's seen and perhaps invisible. While it's normal for all concerned to experience grief and anxiety, remember the healing balm of love and, at times, even gallows humor.

People don't die like we see on TV and in most movies. It's often messier and slower. In truth, there are only two ways to die: suddenly and slowly. Dying fast is usually harder on the survivors, due to unfinished business and questions that can't be answered. Dying slowly is usually harder on the patient, though it takes its toll on all concerned. Pain and suffering can be eased, but rarely can it be removed all together. Worthy of reflection: fifteen percent of all deaths in America are sudden. Eight-five percent of us will die slowly from advanced illness.[1]

An increasingly common death, unique to the hospital's ICU, is called a "compassionate extubation." This transition to comfort measures and the removal of life support happens at a mutually agreed-upon time, by which all have accepted death as inevitable and have said their last goodbyes. While some patients die within minutes, others can hold on for hours and even days, which can feel like forever when we just want the suffering to be over.

Sitting vigil with a dying friend or loved one can be a precious gift and a timeless rite of passage for all concerned. A few things to keep in mind: Consider leaving the bedside now and then, not only to catch your breath, but to allow your loved one the opportunity to die privately, if need be. Some people prefer to be surrounded by loved ones as they're dying. Others prefer to die alone. For people who have been private or independent, their death may come when everyone steps out of the room briefly. Either way, taking a break is important.

Remember that during the dying time, those sitting vigil become the eyes and ears of the clinical team, who usually maintain a respectful distance. Let the team know if they're needed. Feel free to talk or read to your loved one. Consider offering this: "You're safe here, and you're loved." And as hard as it may be to say, "If you need to go, it's okay..." As for personal care, a damp washcloth to gently clean the face and around the mouth can be so welcomed, as can a clean oral swab or lip balm. Remember to leave a door or window cracked open for fresh air. Remember good self-care and to keep breathing fully. This can be a difficult but sacred time for all concerned.

FUNERAL HOMES / BURIAL OPTIONS

Remember friends as you pass by, as you are now so once was I. As I am now soon you must be, prepare yourself to follow me.

—18TH CENTURY EPITAPH

MOST HOSPITALS AND NURSING HOMES will encourage you to take your time after a loved one dies. Time spent viewing the body after death varies from minutes to hours, depending on your needs. After you leave the hospital or nursing home, the body will be cleaned, normally placed in a body bag, and transferred to a morgue to await pickup by a funeral home or cremation provider. If you or your loved ones would like to clean or anoint the deceased, just ask your nurse. Usually, it can be arranged. If death occurs at home under hospice care, a member of the team will be on-call to visit and "pronounce" the death. Wait to call the undertaker until each person has had enough time to say goodbye.

In choosing a funeral home, it's okay to shop around. Call two or three providers. Be sure to compare apples to apples: Do you want to pursue a cremation or a burial? To view or not? To have a gathering or not? Being an informed consumer can mean the difference between feeling satisfied and feeling taken advantage of. Most funeral providers I've worked with are ethical people providing an essential service.

As a growing number of people choose to die at home, more personalized, "do it yourself" home funerals are finding their way into the mainstream. Families are once again learning about these traditional tasks from death midwives or death doulas. This might mean keeping the body at home for a time in wake, transporting the corpse to a crematorium, or, in some cases, performing a home burial. The Home Funeral Alliance is an excellent online resource. See their link in the Appendices. Please note that the laws governing after-death care vary greatly from state to state.

GRIEF AND MOURNING

MOURNING IS BEST DESCRIBED as the outward expression of one's grief. Attending a funeral, wearing black, shedding tears at the graveside, and sharing loving memories with family and friends over a meal are all in the name of mourning. A period of mourning, be it formal or informal, usually passes quicker than our grief.

Grief is the universal and normal human response to loss and change. Everyone grieves differently and many people find grieving more difficult than expected. The death of a loved one is like a deep wound that takes time and tender care to heal. The more deeply connected we are to who or what we've lost, the deeper our grief. It's important to take the time needed to grieve fully.

Our grief will wait patiently until we're ready to attend to it. Some of us put off grieving for a long time. Often grief gets buried beneath subsequent losses, which can lead to complications and prolonged sadness. Be willing to grieve and be wary of anyone who suggests that you just "get over it." Our grief is indelibly connected to our love. If we keep loving the ones who have gone ahead of us, there will continue to be an emotional and spiritual connection and, as a result, times of tender grief.

The more traumatic or conflicted the death, the more complicated and time-consuming the grief. A sudden, unexpected death brings the most lingering grief. One of the hardest losses of all, for the loved ones left behind, is when someone takes their own life. Having a trusted friend to accompany us in our grief—not to fix or advise but just to walk with us and bear witness—can make all the difference. Grief can be a profound and humbling teacher. It can be some of the hardest work we ever do. Remember to take breaks. A prevailing truth: The only way out is through.

There is an unmistakable pattern in the varying levels of grief between families and individuals who chose to prepare for the end of life compared to those who do not. Families who talk and prepare still grieve, but their path of grief is generally more straightforward and manageable. Those who, for whatever reasons choose not to plan or to "just see what happens," tend to travel a harder road.

If you have a healthcare agent, please have a more detailed conversation with them given what you're learning. If nothing else, thank them for their willingness. No agent yet? I encourage you to talk with a trusted friend or family member to explore possibilities. You can also talk with your primary care doctor for guidance. As a last resort, there are agencies that will serve in this capacity for a reasonable fee. Google: "Find a legal guardian."

CONCLUSION: TO DIE AS WE WILL

ARCHIMEDES WAS A GREEK MATHEMATICIAN, physicist, engineer, and inventor. In his brilliance, he understood that a simple lever could lift a small rock from a hole and that, theoretically, if the lever was long enough, it could move the world. The systems to which we are beholden can often appear too large to budge. However, we are each a unique point of leverage within those systems, whether it be healthcare, hospital, family, or the inner workings of our own hearts and minds. What is "the world" if not our individual perception and interpretation of it? As we each become more knowledgeable, aware, and empowered to advocate for ourselves, not only do we see life differently, we learn that systems will often shift to accommodate our will.

Over the next twenty years, seventy million boomers will be encountering the life and death issues raised above. The cumulative impact of this generation's choices, often referred to as a Silver Tsunami, will land on healthcare's shore and irrevocably alter the landscape, redefining business as usual. To read this book and to be proactive is to be part of the solution, rather than part of the problem.

Individually, the fulcrum or pivot point is a growing willingness to face and accept the nature of living and dying. It is the dawning realization that to embrace these truths, to talk about them and to plan accordingly, is a gift to ourselves and those who love us. These straightforward remedies can be medicine for the soul and bring peace of mind to lighten the load. Culturally, the pivot point is the boomers' penchant for being informed, finding their voice, and courageously exploring the frontier, while becoming agents of change.

The culmination of change and loss over the course of a lifetime can be a heavy load. Physically, the burden of pain and loss of strength, combined with a loss of mobility and clarity of mind, can be overwhelming. Mentally and emotionally, these cumulative losses can bring waves of debilitating grief, depression, numbness, and confusion. Spiritually, to lose or question one's faith is not unusual. The dark night of the soul is real. So too the valley of the shadow of death. These metaphors resonate on a deep level because they speak to the human experience.

Still, I believe that there is a source of resilience within each of us—call it a light—that shines perpetually. No matter the time or place, there shines a beacon of truth, supporting life, the end of life, and reintegration. From dust we came and to dust we shall return. Recycling is the essence of it. Remembering this helps me be less afraid. When it comes time, let me be ready to cross over the dunes, to realize that all is in its rightful place, to lie down, to surrender, and to return—as a wave slipping back into the sea.

* * *

Appendices

Appendices

FOR CLINICIANS

People die only once. They have no experience to draw on. They need doctors and nurses who are willing to have the hard discussions and say what they have seen, who will help people prepare for what is to come—and escape a warehoused oblivion that few really want.

—Dr. Atul Gawande

Healing is the central goal of life. I'm not speaking of physical healing; a person can die healed. What I mean by healing is a shift in our quality of life away from anguish and suffering toward an experience of integrity, wholeness and inner peace.

—Dr. Balfour Mount

To those of you involved in healthcare, particularly in end-of-life care, thank you for taking the time to read this book. I imagine that much of it is familiar to you. I've added this section because chaplains sometimes get an earful from patients about their doctors, nurses, and clinicians. Most of it is very positive, but I've been asked to pass along a few requests.

Patients and family members are asking for clearer communication from their clinicians. I know this requires an investment of time, which is already in short supply. I believe the call is for better quality communication rather than for quantity. Please remember that our patients are often overwhelmed, perhaps numb, and therefore have a limited attention span. A powerful invitation: "Please let me know what you want so that I can help you."

People have goals and priorities besides living longer. Asking and learning about these priorities empowers us to provide better care, no matter our specialty. Patients also want the truth about prognosis, though the tone and timing of its delivery is important. Please trust that you will not harm your patient by talking about end-of-life issues. In fact, most patients will be relieved you brought it up. Anxiety is normal for both patient and clinician during these discussions. Please don't let this anxiety keep you from the Conversation. To repeat the North Star questions: "What's most important to you right now?" and "How can I help?"

Consider taking advantage of excellent communication resources for clinicians, especially when it comes to the art of sharing a prognosis. In case you're not familiar with it, Ariadne Lab's Serious Illness Conversation Guide is a gold standard resource (see page 156). In addition, the doctors who founded Vital Talk (see page 161) have created important teaching tools to help clinicians be more aware of and address their patient's emotional well-being. Clear communication and collaborative decision-making can make a measurable difference as patients move through the care continuum. For doctors who recognize this need but "don't have enough time," please consider asking a trusted colleague to follow up in your place.

BASIC PRINCIPLES FOR CLINICIANS TO IMPROVE END-OF-LIFE COMMUNICATION

- With essential information, consider writing it down for the patient and family.

- Provide prognostic information as a range; acknowledge uncertainty, e.g., "We think you have several weeks to a few months, but it could be shorter or longer."

- Allow for pauses and silence.

- Listen at least half the time.

- Acknowledge and explore patients' strong emotions.

- Be careful to limit information in response to patients' emotions.

- Avoid focusing solely on medical procedures and overusing medical terminology.

- Focus instead on the patient's quality of life, goals, fears, and concerns.

- Use plain English, and an interpreter, if need be, speaking clearly and slowly, ideally from a seated position.

- Strive to document and exchange information about patients' values and goals while charting and reporting to your team. By understanding and embracing the general ethos of palliative care, every clinician can choose to provide meaningful, patient-led care. Thank you.

"ROLE PLAYS" FOR PATIENTS AND FAMILY TO FURTHER THE CONVERSATION

"Be informed, prepared, polite and persistent"
—DR. IRA BYOCK

(WITH PRIMARY CARE) "Nurse, when I see the doctor next, I'd like to have enough time to discuss my Advance Directive. Can you please make sure that happens? Thanks."

(WITH PRIMARY CARE OR SPECIALIST) "Doctor, I know that my illness makes it difficult to predict when complications might occur. However, could we please talk about what I might expect as my illness progresses? Both best case and worst-case scenarios?"

(WITH PRIMARY CARE OR SPECIALIST) "Doctor, given what we've discussed, would you be willing to help me complete a POLST document?"

WITH ANY TOPIC THAT'S STILL UNCLEAR OR REQUIRES MORE DETAIL: "I'm finding this hard to get my head around. Could you please say that again?"

Sometimes it can be difficult to get our family member(s) or agent's attention. Here are some prompts:

"I need your help with something. Even though I'm OK right now, I'm worried that _____, and I want to be prepared. Can we talk about some things that are important to me?"[1]

"What if something serious or even life threatening happens to me? Do you know what kind of care I'd want? And what I'd expect you to do? Please let me tell you..."

If their reply is something like, "It upsets me when you talk that way," a good response would be: "I know, it upsets me too. But it's important to me." If you're still met with resistance, ask for a commitment to talk soon. Otherwise, consider that there may be a more appropriate agent.

When finishing up an important conversation, to ensure that everyone's on the same page, consider asking for a recap such as: "We've gone over a lot. Let's recap what we've agreed on."

"Doctor, what do you think our loved one's quality of life will be going forward? 'Both best case and worst-case scenarios?"

"Doctor, if this was your mother/father/spouse, what would you do?"

"Doctor, could you please go over that again in simpler language? Thanks."

"Doctor, given everything we know about our loved one, they would want..."

"Doctor, as a loving family, we feel it's important to..."

"Doctor, we need a little more time to come to terms with everything that you've told us. Thanks."

When clinicians offer differing opinions, see if you can meet with them together. At the very least, tell each one that you've received varying opinions and would like help understanding the difference.[2]

ARE SOME CONDITIONS WORSE THAN DEATH?

What would you want in the situations below if treatment would not reverse or improve your condition?

Circle the number from 1 to 5 that best indicates how you feel about these situations. The Key:

1—Definitely want treatments that would keep me alive

2—Probably want treatments that would keep me alive

3—Unsure of what I'd want

4—Probably would NOT want treatments that would keep me alive

5—Definitely do NOT want treatments that would keep me alive

If I can no longer walk but I can get around in a wheelchair

1   2   3   4   5

If I can no longer get outside—I spend all day in the house

1   2   3   4   5

If I can no longer contribute to my family's well-being

1   2   3   4   5

If I'm in severe pain most of the time

    1   2   3   4   5

If I'm in severe discomfort most of the time
(nausea, diarrhea)

    1   2   3   4   5

If I'm on a feeding tube to stay alive

    1   2   3   4   5

If I'm on a kidney dialysis machine to keep me alive

    1   2   3   4   5

If I'm on a breathing machine to keep me alive

    1   2   3   4   5

If I need someone to take care of me 24 hours a day

    1   2   3   4   5

If I can no longer control my bladder or bowels

    1   2   3   4   5

If I live in a nursing home

    1   2   3   4   5

If I can no longer think or talk clearly

    1   2   3   4   5

If I can no longer recognize my family or friends

1   2   3   4   5

If I need to be sedated to control my pain

1   2   3   4   5

THESE ARE THE KIND OF CIRCUMSTANCES that people struggle to come to terms with. Ideally, discuss them with your agent and/or loved ones. If it's too hard to do or not possible, answer the questions and send the list to your agent. They can be added to your advance directive. starttheconversationvt.org

10 STEPS TO START OR RESUME THE CONVERSATION[3]

1. Start where you are. Hopefully you have enough time to proceed gradually. Take it one step at a time. Since you're reading these words, you've already begun to lay the groundwork.

2. Before talking to anyone, it may help to gather your thoughts, perhaps by writing down what you're hoping to ask or convey.

3. There is no "right way" to start the conversation. Hopefully it will unfold naturally, perhaps even humorously. Trust yourself and the people that you'll be talking with. It's all about what works best for you.

4. Think about certain situations that could arise regarding advanced illness.

5. Be willing to discuss these situations, and any related fears or concerns.

6. You don't have to talk about everything in the first conversation. It's a process that hopefully leads to choosing an agent and having a clear understanding with them of what's important to you.

7. Try finishing this sentence: "What matters to me through the end of my life is..." Be prepared to share this.

8. Nothing you say needs to be permanent. You can change your mind as need be.

9. Now that you've started the conversation, keep going. The more willing you are to talk, the better your family and friends will understand what matters to you.

10. If you meet resistance, which is normal, seek to understand the person's reservations. Try to reassure them and explain why this is important to you.

10 STEPS TO UNDERSTAND AND COMPLETE AN ADVANCE DIRECTIVE

1. The Patient Self-Determination Act considers completing an Advance Directive a Right and a Responsibility.

2. Your Advance Directive allows you to communicate your goals of care if you can no longer speak or think clearly. It provides clear guidance to those who care for you.

3. Take time to reflect on what's most important to you; your values, goals, and preferences.

4. If you have a serious or pre-existing condition, learn about both the best case and worst-case outcomes.

5. Who would be the ideal person to serve as your Healthcare Agent, spokesperson and advocate? Ask for their help.

6. Take the time to have a series of in-depth conversations with this person about what's most important to you.

7. Ask for an Advance Directive from your doctor or hospitalist. Or download one from the internet that's approved in your state. Or follow the link for *Five Wishes* on page 157.

8. Carefully review and complete the form, ideally with your Agent. Ask questions of your medical team as needed.

9. The form will need to be witnessed and signed. Most states do not require notarization. Make copies of the completed document for yourself and others.

10. Send or deliver the document to the following: Your Agent, your primary care doctor, and your nearest hospital or hospital of choice. Well done!

CONTINUE THE CONVERSATION IN YOUR COMMUNITY

Are you part of a book club? The sections, *For Further Conversation* after each chapter in this book are designed for individual AND group discussion.

I recommend Michael Hebb's *Let's Talk About Death (over Dinner)*, which encourages people to gather around a dinner table to talk about death. Hebb estimates that since 2013, more than 100,000 "death over dinners" have been held in thirty countries. "How we end our lives is the most important and costly conversation America is not having." From the website: deathoverdinner.org

Also recommended: Jon Underwood's "Death Cafe," where people drink tea, eat cake, and discuss death. The aim is to increase awareness of death to help people make the most of their (finite) lives. To date over 12,000 "Cafe's" have been hosted in 79 countries. deathcafe.com

As midwives attend to birth, Death Doulas are trained to provide support and guidance prior to and after death. Consider contacting a Death Doula in your area: inelda.org or doulagivers.com

Contact your local Hospice Agency and ask about becoming a Hospice Volunteer. To be welcomed and needed in the home of a hospice patient can be a humbling privilege. The Volunteer training and orientation can be of great benefit, whether you become an active volunteer or not.

ADDITIONAL RESOURCES
(LISTED ALPHABETICALLY)

ARIADNE LABS
ariadnelabs.org

"Ariadne Labs is a joint center for health systems innovation at Brigham and Women's Hospital and Harvard T.H. Chan School of Public Health. Our mission is to save lives and reduce suffering by creating scalable solutions that improve health care delivery at the most critical moments for people everywhere." —From the website

CENTER TO ADVANCE PALLIATIVE CARE
getpalliativecare.org

"The Center to Advance Palliative Care (CAPC) is a national organization dedicated to increasing the availability of quality health care for people living with a serious illness. As the nation's leading resource in its field, CAPC provides health care professionals and organizations with the training, tools, and technical assistance necessary to effectively meet this need." —From the website

THE COALITION TO TRANSFORM ADVANCED CARE (C-TAC)
thectac.org

"Our Mission: The Coalition to Transform Advanced Care (C-TAC) is dedicated to the goal that all Americans with serious illness, especially the sickest and most vulnerable, receive comprehensive, high quality, person and family-centered care that is consistent with their goals and values and honors their dignity. We will achieve this by empowering consumers, changing the health delivery system, improving public and private policies, and enhancing provider capacity." —From the website

THE CONVERSATION PROJECT
theconversationproject.org

"The Conversation Project is a public engagement initiative with a goal that is both simple and transformative: to help everyone talk about their wishes for care through the end of life, so those wishes can be understood and respected. We believe that the place for this to begin is at the kitchen table—not in the intensive care unit—with the people who matter most to us before it's too late. All of our materials, including the Conversation Starter Guide, are available to download and print for free." —From the website

FIVE WISHES
fivewishes.org

"Five Wishes is changing the way we talk about advance care planning. It's more than just a document. Five Wishes is a complete approach to discussing and documenting your care and comfort choices. It's about connecting families, communicating with healthcare providers, and showing your community what it means to care for one another."—From the website

HOSPICE SERVICES

Use this link to better understand the core services that all Medicare certified hospice agencies are required to offer: cancer.org/treatment/end-of-life-care/hospice-care/who-provides-hospice-care

KUBLER-ROSS' PHASES OF GRIEF

grief.com

"The five stages are a part of the framework that makes up our learning to live with the one we lost. They are tools to help us frame and identify what we may be feeling. But they are not stops on some linear timeline in grief. Not everyone goes through all of them or in a prescribed order. Our hope is that with these stages comes the knowledge of grief 's terrain, making us better equipped to cope with life and loss. At times, people in grief will often report more stages. Just remember your grief is as unique as you are."—David Kessler, from the website

MASLOW'S HIERARCHY OF NEEDS

verywellmind.com/what-is-maslows-hierarchy-of-needs-4136760

MEDICARE'S HOME HEALTH BENEFIT

medicare.gov

Use this link to view Medicare's official booklet on Home Health Care: medicare.gov/Pubs/pdf/10969-Medicare-and-Home-Health-Care.pdf

NATIONAL HOME FUNERAL ALLIANCE:
homefuneralalliance.org

"To educate families and communities to care for their loved ones after death." —From the website

NATIONAL POLST FORM
polst.org

"There is a National POLST Form, but most states still use their own state version of POLST... POLST forms are medical orders that your provider uses to tell another provider what treatments you want when you cannot speak for yourself. Since the POLST form is how your provider tells another provider what you want, the words and phrases on the form use medical terminology. The POLST form was not created for patients to fill out and complete: your provider should be the person filling it out after talking with you."—From the website

PREPARE
prepareforyourcare.org

"PREPARE is a step-by-step program with video stories to help you: Have a voice in your medical care, talk with your doctors and fill out an advance directive form to put your wishes in writing." —From the website

RESPECTING CHOICES
respectingchoices.org

"Our Mission: Guide organizations and communities worldwide to effectively implement and sustain evidence-based systems that provide person-centered care. Our Vision: Transform healthcare culture by integrating and disseminating best practices to achieve person-centered care. Respecting Choices is a division of the Coalition to Transform Advanced Care (C-TAC)." —From the website

TOTAL PAIN
pallipedia.org/total-pain

VILLAGE-TO-VILLAGE NETWORK
vtvnetwork.org

"What is a Village? Neighbors Caring for Neighbors. Villages are grassroots, community-based organizations formed through a cadre of caring neighbors who want to change the paradigm of aging. Local Villages connect members to a full range of practical support services to help with non-medical household tasks, services, programs, and transportation. Villages also promote staying active by coordinating recreational, social, educational, and cultural programs. These social activities minimize isolation and promote interaction amongst their peers. The Village Movement originated in Boston with Beacon Hill Village, leading the way for a more economically efficient model for aging." —From the website

VITAL TALK
vitaltalk.org

"VitalTalk is the premier training organization for clinicians seeking to advance their communication skills. Just as no doctor is born knowing how to handle a scalpel, the same is true for how to communicate effectively with seriously ill patients and their families. Whether in person or online, clinicians feel safe practicing newly learned skills through VitalTalk's evidenced-based training methodologies using simulated patients, all in a confidential setting. Our vision is that every seriously ill patient will be surrounded by clinicians who can speak about what matters most and match care to values."— From their website

NOTES ON SOURCES

NOTES TO INTRODUCTION

1. under difficult circumstances: "Preferences for Place of Care and Place of Death..." Palliative Medicine 19, no. 6 (2005): 492-99

2. systemic conveyor belt: Jessica Nutik Zitter, MD, *Extreme Measures, Finding a Better Path to the End of Life*, (2017)

3. until it's too late: The Conversation Project, theconversationproject.org

4. seventy-seven years for men: Arias E, Teja-da-Vera B, Ahmad F. Provisional life expectancy estimates for January through June 2020. Vital Statistics Rapid Release; no. 10. Hyattsville, MD: National Center for Health Statistics. February 2021. DOI: https://dx.doi.org/10.15620/cdc:100392.

5. The speaker is Death: www.thestorytelling-resource-centre.com/Appointment_in_Samarra.html

NOTES TO CHAPTER ONE

1. coping with advanced illness: Institute of Medicine. *Dying in America: Improving Quality and Honoring Individual Preferences Near the End of Life*. 2015 Mar 19. 5, Available from:

ncbi.nlm.nih.gov/books/NBK285671/

2. due to medical costs: David U. Himmelstein, Robert M. Lawless, Deborah Thorne, Pamela Foohey, Steffie Woolhandler, "Medical Bankruptcy: Still Common Despite the Affordable Care Act," *American Journal of Public Health* 109, no. 3 (March 1, 2019): pp. 431-433. doi. org/10.2105/AJPH.2018.304901

3. even to many providers: Institute of Medicine. *Dying in America: Improving Quality and Honoring Individual Preferences Near the End of Life.* 2015 Mar 19. 5, Available from: ncbi.nlm.nih.gov/books/NBK285671

4. an intensive care unit stay: Kelley, Amy S et al. "Hospice enrollment saves money for Medicare and improves care quality across a number of different lengths-of-stay." *Health affairs (Project Hope)* vol. 32,3 (2013): 552-61. doi:10.1377/hlthaff.2012.0851

5. places where people die: Atul Gawande, *Being Mortal,* (2014)

6. ibid, 193.

7. over 36 million admissions: American Hospital Association, www.aha.org/system/files/ media/file/2020/01/2020-aha-hospital-fast-facts-new-Jan-2020.pdf

8. sickest and most vulnerable patients: Jessica Nutik Zitter, MD, *Extreme Measures, Finding a Better Path to the End of Life,* (2017)

9. persistently chooses against it: Rachel E. Bernacki, Susan D. Block, for the American College of Physicians High Value Care Task Force. Communication About Serious Illness Care Goals: A Review and Synthesis of Best Practices. JAMA Intern Med.2014;174(12):1994–2003. doi:10.1001/jamainternmed.2014.5271

10. an extended stay: Smith AK, McCarthy E, Weber E, Cenzer IS, Boscardin J, Fisher J, Covinsky K. Half of older Americans seen in emergency department in last month of life; most admitted to hospital, and many die there. Health Aff (Millwood). 2012 June; 31(6):1277-85. doi: 10.1377/hlthaff.2011.0922. Erratum in: Health

11. information about our wishes: Rachel E. Bernacki, Susan D. Block, for the American College of Physicians High Value Care Task Force. Communication About Serious Illness Care Goals: A Review and Synthesis of Best Practices. JAMA Intern Med.2014;174(12):1994–2003. doi:10.1001/jamainternmed.2014.5271

12. higher costs of care: ibid.

13. how much does it cost? ABIM Foundation, Choosing Wisely: abimfoundation.org

14. 33 days before death: Mack JW, Cronin A, Keating NL, et al. Associations between end-of-life discussion characteristics and care received near death: a prospective cohort study. J Clin Oncol. 2012;30 (35):4387-4395.

15. patients with similar illness: ibid.

1. a developmental achievement: *Maslow's Hierarchy of Needs*, A.H. Maslow, "A Theory of Human Motivation," *Psychological Review* 50, (1943)

2. make decisions about their care: Understanding Health Care Decisions at the End of Life, National Institute on Aging, <u>nia.nih.gov/health/understanding-health-care-decisions-end-life</u>

3. completes an advance directive: <u>healthaffairs.org/doi/10.1377/hlthaff.2017.0175</u>

4. an advance directive in place: Bernard J. Hammes, Editor, *Having Your Own Say, Getting the Right Care When It Matters Most*, (2012)

5. anywhere in our country: ibid.

6. regarding their treatment options: Rachel E. Bernacki, Susan D. Block, for the American College of Physicians High Value Care Task Force. *Communication About Serious Illness Care Goals: A Review and Synthesis of Best Practices*. JAMA Intern Med.2014;174(12):1994–2003. doi:10.1001/jamainternmed.2014.5271

NOTES TO CHAPTER THREE

1. not leave the ICU alive: Society of Critical Care Medicine, (2020) sccm.org/Communications/Critical-Care-Statistics

2. is less than 3%: Respecting Choices, Gunderson Health System, (2013)

3. chosen DNR / AND for themselves: Stanford Medicine, med.stanford.edu/news/all-news/2014/05/most-physi-cians-would-forgo-aggressive-treat-ment-for-themselves

NOTES TO CHAPTER FOUR

1. "I love you.": Ira Byock, *The Four Things That Matter Most*, (2004)

2. during serious illness: Torke AM, Sachs GA, Helft PR, et al. Scope and outcomes of surrogate decision making among hospitalized older adults. *JAMA Intern Med.* 2014;174(3):370-377.

3. negative effects are minimized: Rachel E. Bernacki, Susan D. Block, for the American College of Physicians High Value Care Task Force. *Communication About Serious Illness Care Goals: A Review and Synthesis of Best Practices*. JAMA Intern Med.2014;174(12):1994–2003. doi:10.1001/jamainternmed.2014.5271

4. took place after hospitalization: ibid.

5. to cure their cancer: Weeks JC, Catalano PJ, Cronin A, etal. Patients' expectations about effects of chemotherapy for advanced cancer. N. England J Med. 2012; 367(17):1616-1625.

6. goals of care: ibid.

7. under hospice care: statnews. com/2019/12/11/more-americans-die-at-home

8. unacceptable suffering: David S. White, Master's level thesis: *Embodying Compassion Amidst Suffering: Examining the Chaplain's Role In Responding Ethically to those Considering the Voluntary Suspension of Eating and Drinking at End-of-Life*. (2020)

9. ultimate individual right: Symons X., American Nurses Association Endorses VSED. bioedge.org/bioethics/american-nurses-association-endorses-vsed/12430 (2017)

10. truly committed to VSED: Robert C. Macauley, Ethics in Palliative Care, (2018)

NOTES TO CHAPTER FIVE

1. to both patient and family: Hospice Facts and Figures. Alexandria, VA: National Hospice & Palliative Care Organization. August 2020. nhpco.org/hospice-facts-figures.

2. endures all things: *The Bible*. 1 Corinthians 13:7.

1. last 3 months of life: Rachel E. Bernacki, Susan D. Block, for the American College of Physicians High Value Care Task Force. *Communication About Serious Illness Care Goals: A Review and Synthesis of Best Practices*. JAMA Intern Med.2014;174(12):1994–2003. doi:10.1001/jamainternmed.2014.5271

2. live slightly longer: Regnard C. Double effect is a myth leading a double life. BMJ. 2007;334(7591):440. doi:10.1136/bmj.39136.502361.FA

3. however we define it: Richardson P. Spirituality, religion, and palliative care. *Annals of Palliative Care Medicine*.2014;3(3):150-159. doi:10:3978/j.issn.2224-5820.2014.07.05

4. or LSD: Krebs TS, Johansen PØ. Over 30 million psychedelic users in the United States. F1000Res. 2013;2:98. Published 2013 Mar 28. doi:10.12688/f1000research.2-98.v1

1. more than their parents: www.statista.com/statistics/1040079/life-expectancy-united-states-all-time

2. beds, are overflowing: www.cdc.gov/nchs/

fastats/nursing-home-care.htm

3. with the disease: Alzheimer's Association (2021): alz.org/alzheimers-dementia/facts-figures

4. form of dementia: ibid.

5. 1 of 3 are older than 65: ibid.

6. in nursing homes: ibid.

Notes to Chapter Eight

1. is five minutes: nena.org/page/911Statistics

2. leave the facility alive: Bernard J. Hammes, Editor, *Having Your Own Say, Getting the Right Care When It Matters Most*, (2012)

3. to stay alive: Davison SN., *End-of-life Care Preferences and Needs: Perceptions of Patients with Chronic Kidney Disease*. Clin J Am Soc Nephrol. 2010;5(2):195-204.

4. Burger King Restaurants: *Kidney Dialysis Is a Booming Business. Is It Also a Rigged One?* ScientificAmerica.com.(2021)

5. for a fall: Liu SW, Obermeyer Z, Chang Y, Shankar KN. *Frequency of ED Revisits and Death Among Older Adults after a Fall*. Am J Emergency Med. 2015;33(8):1012-1018. doi:10.1016/j.ajem.2015.04.023

6. from a fall: ibid.

7. under similar conditions: National Center for

Health Statistics, www.cdc.gov/nchs/fastats/
nursing-home-care.htm

8. amidst it all: adapted from jackkornfield.com/
meditation-equanimity

Notes to Chapter Nine

1. slowly from advanced illness: Center to Advance Palliative Care (2021): media.capc.org/
filer_public/68/bc/68bc93c7-14ad-4741-9830-
8691729618d0/capc_press-kit.pdf

Notes to Appendices

1. things that are important to me: The Conversation Project, theconversationproject.org
2. understanding the difference: ibid.
3. Or Resume The Conversation: ibid.

ACKNOWLEDGMENTS

It's a profound privilege to accompany patients and their loved ones near the end of life. The "Spiritual Care" badge that I wear throughout the hospital is a passport into a personal and intimate world where life and death rest in the balance. It's often a sobering reality, yet when it comes to touching the heart of what matters most, I've found few settings to rival it. The call to chaplaincy has brought purpose and meaning to my life and has been a saving grace. In addition, I'm grateful to be part of an interdisciplinary team that allows me to collaborate with such gifted colleagues.

I'd like to again recognize the Hospice and Palliative Care Pioneers, and the legions of clinicians, caregivers, and volunteers they've inspired, who bring compassionate care to millions of bedsides each year, the world over.

I'm grateful for my family's loving support, particularly for my brother Netaka's editorial help, and for my mother's spirited conversations over the years about death and dying. And to Sandy, my first wife, who taught me the art of caregiving. And to our son, Freeman, who's innate joy, quiet wisdom, and devoted parenting are a tribute to his mother's legacy.

To Vicki DeArmon, my friend, editor, and muse, "thank you" falls short. And to Alicia Feltman, who created this book from a manuscript and our website from thin air, this project simply would not have happened without you both. Many thanks, as well, to numerous friends and associates who contributed their valuable time and feedback as advance readers. Without exception, your suggestions have made for a better book.

In the end, I want to acknowledge a group of unsung heroes, our schoolteachers. And mine, from Douglas G. Grafflin Elementary through college literature, who patiently taught not only the craft of writing, but the essential value of revision. Thank you, to one and all.

— DSW

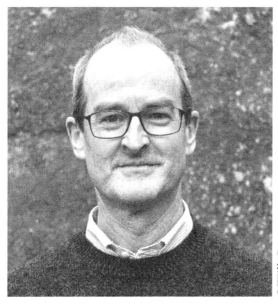

©Will Gray

ABOUT THE AUTHOR

DAVID WHITE works with seriously ill patients and
their family members as a full time, senior chaplain
at Reading Hospital; a 500 bed, Level 1 Trauma
Center in Berks County, PA. Visit him online at
onemillionpledges.com

.

Made in the USA
Monee, IL
29 September 2023

43664113R00121